KU-186-416

For my children
Emma and Robert van der Vliet.
With love and gratitude

BRIEFINGS are short books which explain and clarify complex contemporary subjects, written for the non-specialist by experts in their fields. Themes and topics covered include Education, Cosmology, Medical Ethics, Political Ideology, Structuralism, Quantum Physics and Comparative Religion among others.

CONTENTS

PREFACE

Who gets AIDS and why? There are no simple answers to these questions. Vulnerability lies in a complex interaction of environment, behaviour, medical and social circumstances. This Briefing explains how, in plagues of the past like the Black Death, the current AIDS pandemic and pandemics yet to come, similar factors are at work – environmental change, population growth, social upheaval and migration, urbanization, poverty, discrimination and prejudice, gender inequality and religious, medical and sexual beliefs and practices. In its reflection of power relationships, from the interpersonal to the international, AIDS provides a potent lens through which to view the human condition.

In the ten years I have brooded over this book, many people have, with or without their knowledge, played a formative role in its structure. I would especially like to thank Professor John Moodie, head of the Department of Virology, University of Cape Town, who asked the questions for which I hope this book provides some answers. Thanks are also due to Malcolm Steinberg, Andre Jaquet and Mamphela Ramphele (South Africa), Pat Duggan (Canberra), Gillian Hawley (Cambridge), Uwe Leonardy and Martina Schoeps-Potthoff (Bonn), Jacques du Guerny, and Daniela Colombo and the AIDoS Association (Rome), Gustaaf Wolvaardt (Geneva), Stefano Bertozzi, Ben Nkowane, Dorothy Blake and Tony Burton (WHO, Geneva), François Wasserfallen (Bern) and Douglas Feldman (Florida, USA).

i

More immediately I would like to thank my husband, David Welsh, for encouragement and painstaking proof-reading, and Emma van der Vliet for her unswerving belief that I would eventually produce the thing!

My special thanks to Cathy Welsh who intelligently and uncomplainingly translated my pencilled drafts into a respectable manuscript. For someone computer illiterate, the technical support of Robert van der Vliet and Simon Welsh has also been very reassuring.

The enthusiasm of Peter Collins, series editor of Briefings and Robert Dudley of Bowerdean Publishing has been invaluable in ensuring that the book was written at all.

Cape Town
September 1995

INTRODUCTION

AIDS is here to stay. It is like the day after Hiroshima.
The world has changed and will never be the same
again.

Dr June Osborn (1988:445)

The 1960s and early 1970s were years of convulsive social change. They saw the end of empires, the growth of cities, secularization, the global village. A chain of 'utopian eruptions' (Berger 1986:223) characterized the times. Colonies gained independence and set off, full of hope, down the path of modernization and development. The civil rights movement in the United States promised equality to black Americans and in turn helped fuel liberation movements for women and homosexuals. Nothing of the old order seemed permanent or sacred. God was declared dead. Patriotism was discredited in the clamour against the Vietnam war, and marriage and the family buckled under the onslaught of rising divorce rates, single parenting, abortion reforms and the feminist movement.

It was against this turbulent background, that love was pronounced 'free'. Objectively, First World sexual activity did seem to carry a lower price tag than at any other time in human history. Antibiotics cured its diseases, contraceptives prevented the pregnancies, modern

1

antenatal care and obstetrics made childbirth – for those who still wanted it – safe.

The first suggestion that the pronouncement was premature, even among the world's most affluent people, came with the genital herpes scare. First reported in the mid-1970s, estimated infections in the United States were as high as twenty million a decade later, with half a million new infections annually. Although it was incurable, it was painful and inconvenient rather than fatal. By July 1980, *Time* magazine had dubbed it 'the new sexual leprosy'. It was seen as the wages of the era's sexual sins. Like the wave of syphilis and gonorrhoea which had accompanied the social upheavals at the beginning of this century – urbanization, industrialization, immigration and changing family patterns – herpes became a metaphor for the sickness of society itself. (Brandt 1987)

Herpes and its significance were undoubtedly blown out of proportion by the media. The AIDS pandemic was another story. Here was a disease that was actually lethal and spreading at great speed in the very communities that symbolized the changing world. By the time the first cases were identified in the USA in 1981, the social legacy of the previous two decades was already under attack. The speed of transformation unnerved people. A new conservatism, epitomized by the governments of Ronald Reagan and Margaret Thatcher, was demanding a return to 'morality' and 'family values'. Far more than the relatively minor symptoms of herpes, the physical corruption of AIDS, as Susan Sontag pointed out, matched our image of growing social and environmental corruption. AIDS reinforced our 'end-of-era feeling', (1989:78) 'the countdown to a millennium' and the 'rise of apocalyptic thinking.' (1989:87)

2

Introduction

AIDS, like other epidemic diseases before it, thrived because the circumstances were right. As we shall see in Chapter 1, epidemics require a particular ecology, an interaction of environmental and social conditions which allow for the rapid transmission of the disease-causing organism. The 1960s and 1970s had provided these conditions. They had also created unease and insecurity, a feeling of loss of control in the face of rapid change. AIDS was both a product of and a metaphor for the times. Like Hiroshima, AIDS changed the way we saw the world. Writers have tried to persuade us that AIDS is a natural phenomenon, that it has no moral meaning, that there is no message in its spread. (Sontag 1989:86) People seldom experience epidemics as purely natural phenomena. The AIDS epidemic drew its meaning not only from the times in which it arrived, but also from those who became infected.

Cruelly, the disease surfaced first among those already marginalized and stigmatized, living 'symptoms' of our troubled times – the gay community, injecting drug users and poor minority communities. When it appeared in Africa it became part of what Ann Larson has called the media's 'African disaster' obsession, portraying a continent facing 'insurmountable calamities', rather than 'problems with social and political causes'. (Larson 1990:5) In subsequent years, AIDS was to spread to virtually every corner of the earth. As its significance and its threat were realized, in each place the disease was given a 'social construction' – it assimilated the meanings, the anxieties and the prejudices of that time and place. In the United States fears of changing sexual mores allowed homophobia to re-emerge as a fear of AIDS. In France and elsewhere in Europe, threats of job losses to waves of new immigrants revived old xenophobic attitudes, this time in the guise of fears about foreigners bringing AIDS into the country. In South Africa, fears of a new social order reactivated racism masquerading as concerns about AIDS in desegregated swimming pools and lavatories.

3

AIDS was seen as divine retribution, punishment for immorality, an answer to the over-population problem. AIDS vindicated conservatism.

Initial assertions by individuals, communities or states that AIDS did not concern them, or would not become a problem, because they were not gay, or atheist, or capitalist, or black, gave way to the realization that nobody, and no society, was immune. By 1991, the World Health Organization's (WHO) Global Programme on AIDS, had reports of AIDS in 163 countries, and AIDS became a formal political issue everywhere. Health budgets had to take blood testing and patient care into account; changes to immigration laws were debated; foreign aid packages, to enable developing countries to cope with the burden, were negotiated.

These issues, though, were just the calm and measured face of public policy. In fact, AIDS was to be at every level a 'political' issue, and an issue that inspired the most anguished and vitriolic debates. For the purposes of this book, 'politics' will refer not only to formal and institutional politics, but also to the strategizing that underlies social behaviour and alignments. It will examine the politics of AIDS in terms of the power relationships inherent in all human acts, most centrally here the power to control and influence people, events and resources.

The tension between those 'in control', and those infected or at risk, and the way in which their relative power and influence affects policy and responses – the interplay of power and powerlessness – will to a significant extent shape the emerging pandemic. Power lies not just in the overt, public realm where, for instance, public health policies dealing with AIDS, are debated in a political forum. It lies also in the extent to which individuals or groups are aware of the risks or are able to get their agenda on the table for debate in the first place; in their leverage within the social system; in their wilful resistance to the messages; in the sanctions which can be used against them if they push for unpopular measures. There is power, too, in the deliberate politicization of the AIDS issue, in the way in which perceptions of risk can be manipulated for political advantage by individuals or groups.

Chapter 2 will examine the power that comes from control over and access to resources, constituencies and policy making. To exercise such power, one must enter dangerous terrain, for AIDS is a minefield of issues that could easily blow up in one's face. Foreign donors find themselves trapped in internecine battles between governments and non-governmental organizations (NGOs) fighting for control of funds; NGOs fight amongst themselves for the funds which would enable them to extend patronage. Information and knowledge are passed on or withheld to further political ambitions or discredit political opponents. Medical care and new drugs become items of contest and conflict. Policy issues, directly connected with AIDS such as sex education in schools or the rights of HIV-positive workers to retain employment, or issues indirectly believed to be associated with AIDS, such as gays in the military, are no longer simply items for rational debate. Everywhere the fate of AIDS programmes seem to teeter on the knife-edge of politics.

AIDS becomes grist to the political mill. It is an issue around which to build a constituency by determining, articulating and protecting the rights of a particular group, or extending patronage. Where a strong and honest AIDS policy might alienate a constituency, political considerations might favour judicious lying or evasion of the issues.

Power exists always in counterpoint to powerlessness. Both are relative terms – no one has absolute power in any human situation. The way the disease, and those with HIV or AIDS are perceived will affect their ability to cope. Marginalizing or blaming the infected disempowers them. Even the use of the term 'AIDS victims' is a factor; sufferers reject it in favour of the term People with AIDS (PWAs). Rather than helpless, powerless 'victims', PWAs see themselves as agents, working with whatever medical, psychological or political tools they have available, to improve their chances and their situation. People who are HIV-positive talk of the way the diagnosis shunts them into a category of the 'un-dead', a 'vampire' status, and the need to claim back their lives, to be seen as living with HIV, rather than dying of AIDS, for what could be years of healthy asymptomatic life. As Brazilian PWA Herbert Daniel proclaims: "I'm alive; all this talk about my death is an outright lie." (Daniel and Parker 1993:140)

Chapter 3 deals with this process of 'disease construction' – the explanatory model which evolves to fit the way people perceive the disease in relation to who is infected. How the disease is constructed in the public mind will profoundly influence the relative powerlessness of the infected. The early association of the disease with socially and politically marginalized groups, who, as we have seen, had come to be associated with the social disruption and decay of turbulent times, rekindled old prejudices and discrimination. Gays, blacks, drug users, Haitians, immigrants, Africans were the objects of a new bigotry – they were 'high-risk groups'. The fact that it was not group membership but a particular personal behaviour pattern that put people at risk, was ignored.

Gays in places as far apart as San Francisco, New York, Europe and Latin America became the victims of gay bashing; in Egypt, Cyprus and China, to name a few out of many countries, black African students and tourists found themselves singled out for HIV testing to be allowed entry to the countries. Personal behaviour would be irrelevant; their visibility made them handy scapegoats for people's fears and prejudices. The legacies of racism and homophobia, and the empowerment which followed gay liberation have shaped responses to the epidemic; they are the focus of Chapter 3.

Chapter 4 examines the role of socio-economic conditions in precipitating the AIDS crisis. There can be no doubt that poverty, war, migrations, drought, famine, poor health status and health care and particularly the oppression and brutalization of women and children all interact with the virus, and assist it to spread, by accelerating interaction, lowering physical resistance to infection or destroying the normative systems that made for sexual conservatism. The problem with seeing AIDS as essentially a product of poverty and socio-economic conditions is that prevention and cure must then be postponed till Utopia – or something approaching it. While promising this Utopia might be a politically useful position for politicians to adopt – enabling them to score points against their opponents for not attaining it – it is hardly an empowering strategy for their followers. To suggest that only a changed social and economic order can deliver them from disease, is to take from them their opportunities to protect themselves, to develop strategies for coping despite poverty. Long term, socio-economic upliftment may well curb the epidemic, but AIDS is happening in the short term. Leaders are needed who can enable people and communities to devise appropriate strategies for coping with AIDS, rather than using it as a political football.

The issue is part of the wider conflict centering on ideas of 'blame'. Who is to blame for the epidemic? Is it the victim, who became infected because of his or her behaviour – thus absolving the state or social institutions from responsibility for creating social conditions in which AIDS flourishes? Or are the state, the 'system' and social institutions to blame – thereby exculpating the individual? These mutually contradictory positions provide the battlegrounds for much of AIDS politics. The truths and realities must lie somewhere in between, differently located for every community in time and place, an interaction of personal behaviour and socio-economic circumstances. To simply blame one or the other in the way some politicians, or demagogues, or religious leaders have done, is to make rational responses and policies impossible. It is playing with fire, and we all stand to be burned.

The AIDS epidemic is still very new. Relative to the Black Death which came and went within a few years or the 1918–1919 influenza which was over in a few months, it has already had a long life for an epidemic, but AIDS is a 'long-wave' epidemic. The extended asymptomatic latency period – one of its more diabolical features – means that people who have become infected while you were reading this introduction will only become ill years from now, in the meantime possibly infecting a whole web of others. For a new epidemic, it has taught us a lot. Most discouragingly, perhaps, it has demonstrated that while medicine has made giant strides, human beings remain trapped in behaviour and thinking we would like to believe went out with the Dark Ages. We have been, and will be, witnesses to immense suffering and hardship.

Nevertheless, the fight against AIDS has had some positive outcomes, as Chapter 5 suggests. It has humbled a generation which believed that it had microbes beaten and made us battle-ready for what will undoubtedly be new diseases yet to come. The very ferocity of the onslaught has brought some measure of scientific openness and collaboration – and some major advances that will help us in our fight against other diseases. It has demonstrated that communities under threat, be they the gay men of the United States or impoverished peasants in Uganda, can come up with innovative coping strategies, which governments and NGOs, would do well to emulate, rather than indulge in endless – and expensive – re-inventions of the wheel. It has opened up whole

8

areas as diverse as law, medicine, religion, morality, ethics, and international relations to heated public debate. As Osborn says, the world will never be the same again.

CHAPTER ONE

TIMES OF PLAGUE: EPIDEMICS IN PERSPECTIVE

The plague not only depopulates and kills, it gnaws the moral stamina and frequently destroys it entirely ... Times of plague are always those in which the bestial and the diabolical side of human nature gains the upper hand.

Barthold Niebuhr, 1816 (in Nohl, J 1961: Preface)

Ever since we turned from hunting and gathering to crop growing and the denser settlements and burgeoning populations this allowed, 'times of plague' have probably been part of the human lot. Contemporary records dating back as far as the thirteenth century BC in China and 2000 BC in the Middle East, chronicle the way towns, nations or even the world at large were periodically plunged into misery and death by diseases for which the medical knowledge of the day had no answer. (McNeill 1985) To ordinary people, caught in their path, the sudden appearance of epidemic diseases was terrifying and inexplicable. They were seen as punishment for sin, the work of sorcerers or witches, apocalyptic messengers of the end of the world. Where science and reason provided no explanations or solutions, people turned to supernatural beliefs and superstitions, to blame and victimization to help them cope with the unknown.

Epidemics are not merely medical phenomena. They have their roots in social conditions, and major epidemics can in turn profoundly affect how societies evolve. Smallpox, introduced into Mexico by an infected Spanish sailor in 1520, raged through the Indian populations of Central and South America killing between 15 and 18 million of the estimated 25 million native people. (Swenson 1989:18) For the Spanish, with a natural immunity born of long historical exposure, the epidemic proved a most potent ally in the subsequent conquest of the Americas. As McNeill commented:

> there could be no doubt about which side of the struggle enjoyed divine favour. The religions, priesthoods, and way of life built around the old Indian Gods could not survive such a demonstration of the superior power of the God the Spaniards worshipped. Little wonder, then, that the Indians accepted Christianity and submitted to Spanish control so meekly.
> (McNeill 1985:10)

For Europeans the epidemic which most fundamentally affected their society was probably the great plague, or 'Black Death' of the fourteenth century. Barbara Tuchman's study of the 'calamitous fourteenth century' gives a graphic account of the plague and its aftermath. Originating in China, it moved across central Asia and India to Europe via the trade routes. Between 1347, when trading-ships arrived in Sicily 'with dead and dying men at the oars' (Tuchman 1987:92) to

1350, when it had run its course in Europe, 'a third of the world died'. (ibid.: 94) The loss of 25 million people was to have profound and permanent effects on Europe.

Contemporary writers describe scenes of carnage: of mass burial pits overflowing, of piles of bodies left on the streets to be collected by plague carts for anonymous disposal, of parents deserting infected children and children fleeing from their dying parents, of the victims dying in terror without the benefit of confession or last rites, because there were not enough priests to attend them, especially since many had fled or themselves succumbed to the epidemic. Tuchman writes: 'the plague was not the kind of calamity that inspired mutual help. Its loathsomeness and deadliness did not herd people together in mutual distress but only prompted their desire to escape each other.' (ibid.: 96)

Nowhere was the inhumanity of the time more obvious than in the treatment of Jews. In its search for a scapegoat to blame for the epidemic, Europe picked the Jews. This antagonism had ancient roots. Deprived of their civil rights for centuries, the Jews had been portrayed as fiends intent on destroying the human race since the Crusades, and even before. Their social and economic persecution grew throughout the twelth and thirteenth centuries; by 1346, the Jews were ready-made targets.

Tuchman writes: 'While Divine punishment was accepted as the plague's source, people in their misery still looked for a human agent upon whom to vent the hostility that could not be vented on God.' (ibid.: 109) 'Confessions', extracted under torture, revealed an international Jewish conspiracy – rabbinical instructions to poison Europe's wells and springs with the intention of destroying Christendom and establishing Jewish control over the world. Papal attempts to control the hysteria, pointing out that Jews, too, fell victim to the plague or that it raged in places where there were no Jews to poison wells, were fruit-less. In Basle, in January 1349, several hundred Jews were burned in 'a wooden house especially constructed for the purpose on an island in the Rhine, and a decree was passed that no Jews should be allowed to settle in Basle for 200 years.' (ibid.:113) In Strasbourg, in February 1349, even before the plague had reached the city, its 2000-strong Jewish community was herded out to the burial ground 'where all except those who accepted conversion were burned at rows of stakes erected to receive them.' (ibid.:114)

Hysteria, too, was evident in the rapid progress across Europe of the flagellants' movements. Believing the plague to be God's punishment for human sin, the movement, which pre-dated the plague, literally whipped itself into a frenzy in an attempt to emulate the scourging of Christ and his expiation of the sins of the world. Interceding with God on behalf of plague-embattled humanity as they marched from city to city, whipping themselves, they also unwittingly helped spread infec-tion. Worse still, as Tuchman records: 'In every town they entered, the flagellants rushed for the Jewish quarter, trailed by citizens howling for revenge upon the 'poisoners of the wells'.' (ibid.:115) In scenes grim-ly presaging times to come, Jews were slaughtered in their tens of thousands. She records that by the time church and state were willing to act against the flagellants, banning the movement and executing those who did not manage to vanish, 'like night phantoms or mocking ghosts,' (ibid.:116) Western Europe had virtually destroyed its Jewish communities, and reinforced a malevolent stereotype of the Jews which was to have tragic consequences for centuries to come.

The effects of the plague were felt in every aspect of European life. Recurrences of plague over the next 150 years kept the European pop-ulation at its reduced level. (Swenson 1989:17) Some areas had been little affected, others totally depopulated. In a description reminiscent

13

of reports filtering in from African areas hard hit by AIDS today, Tuchman writes: 'When the last survivors, too few to carry on, moved away, a deserted village sank back into the wilderness and disappeared from the map altogether, leaving only a grass-covered ghostly outline to show where mortals once had lived.' (ibid.:95)

The drop in population meant a shortage of labour, and real wages rose dramatically. A ploughman in England who had earned two shillings a week in 1347, received seven shillings in 1349 and ten shillings and sixpence by 1350. Day labourers received not only higher wages, but also lunches of meat pies and ale. At the same time land depopulation meant peasants could move more freely, and the price of livestock, in the absence of cowherds and shepherds, plummeted. (Gottfried 1983:94) For the landholders, the drop in the value of their land and produce, the rise in wages and the shortage of labour directly undermined the old manorial system and marked a shift to modern contractual relationships. (Gottfried 1983:94–95, Swenson 1989:17, Dols 1977:283)

Religious institutions, too, were greatly changed in the plague's aftermath. Death on such a scale, wiping out sinners and saints with equal, undiscriminating brutality numbed people to the religious teachings by which they ordinarily made sense of mortality. It 'intensified the medieval preoccupation with death, judgement, heaven and hell.' (Gottfried 1983:82) Muslim and Christian alike faced the dilemma of whether they should try to resist the plague, or accept it as the will of God or a judgement on their sins.

The failure of the church to provide medical or spiritual comfort, led many to turn to alternative beliefs. Ecstatic sects, such as the flagellants, and apocalyptic and magical beliefs burgeoned, but there were also initiatives among mainstream believers to take their salvation into

14

their own hands with good works, pious acts and pilgrimages that side-lined the formal clergy. (Gottfried 1983:81–88)

The failure of the cleric-physicians to halt the plague, or indeed to save even their own lives, called their medical knowledge into question. The physicians continued to emphasize the immediate cause of the plague as 'pestilential miasma' – a foul air variously believed to emanate from swamps, volcanoes, stars, comets, or even over-population, and spread like wind, mist or smoke across the earth. (Dols 1977:85ff) Nevertheless, speculation grew about the contagious nature of the disease; strict quarantine was enforced in some cities. Tuchman notes that the despotic archbishop of Milan ordered that all the inhabitants of the city's first three houses afflicted by plague, dead, sick or well, were to be immediately walled up in a common tomb. 'Whether or not owing to his promptitude, Milan escaped lightly in the roll of the dead.' (ibid.:108) New secular physicians and medical texts, and rudimentary hospitals and public health measures arose in response to the crisis.

While infected rats and fleas were the immediate cause of the plague, its appearance in the mid-fourteenth century was the result of natural and social conditions originating centuries before. Swenson (1989:16) describes the eleventh and twelfth centuries as relatively disease-free, with political stability, and a dramatic rise in both population and food production. Around AD 1300, mean temperatures in Europe dropped significantly, leading to widespread crop failures. In the famine that followed, peasants (and quite probably rats, too) flocked to the towns. In the poverty, crowding and squalor that ensued, rats and their flea fellow-travellers multiplied rapidly. It also greatly facilitated the spread of the pneumonic form of the disease spread by bacilli sprayed into the air by coughing and sneezing and inhaled by others. (Dols 1977:73) A key piece in the puzzle was the apparent transformation of the plague

15

bacillus, *Pasteurella pestis,* from a relatively innocuous variety endemic in Central Asia, that infected rats, to the virulent form that ravaged Europe. Why – or even whether – this happened is not known, but it was the growing shipping trade with the East that brought the first infected ships' rats to the harbours of Sicily, Genoa and France. All these factors were necessary preconditions for the plague; like epidemics down the centuries, and the AIDS epidemic today, no virus or bacillus alone can create such medical catastrophes.

What can this historical retrospective teach us about the AIDS pandemic we face today? While no two epidemics are the same in causes, courses or consequences, their history leaves markers which we can usefully examine. How individuals, communities, governments respond can offer insights – often disconcerting – that may help us evaluate policies, predict reactions and devise strategies that will save us having to reinvent wheels.

Unlike *Pasteurella pestis,* which had repeatedly afflicted Europe, Asia and the Middle East long before the Black Death (Dols 1977), AIDS, at least in its current virulent epidemic form, appears to be a relatively new disease. Robert Gallo, whose research team played an important role in identifying the human immuno-deficiency virus (HIV) and its role in precipitating AIDS, suggests that HIV 'was possibly, and perhaps probably, due to the microbe's transmission from animal to human and from a remote section of the world to the developed world.' (Gallo 1991:132)

Like *Pasteurella pestis,* HIV has gone on the rampage in a world peculiarly suited to its special needs. The late twentieth century is, as was the fourteenth century in Europe, a time of increasing human interaction, of permeable borders and extensive trade and travel. While the plague depended on infected rats and fleas as the main carriers, it was

16

the traders' caravans and ships which enabled these creatures to travel the enormous distances between isolated places in Central Asia and across the sea to Europe. The HI virus similarly appears to have hitched rides in its human hosts as they jetted between continents, walked from village to village, or rattled back and forth in trucks between city and coast all over the Third World. Nowhere is the 'global village' metaphor more chillingly illustrated than in the speed with which AIDS encircled the planet.

Urban life, with its dense social networks and more elastic sexual norms, provides ideal conditions for the virus. The coincidence of the sexual revolution, gay liberation and the 'fast lane' life of cities such as Los Angeles, San Francisco and New York allowed homosexual men to experiment with lifestyles and sexual relationships which provided for very rapid transmission of the virus. (Shilts 1987) In Africa, South America and increasingly in Asia, the same dense urban social networks and fluid normative systems allowed for patterns of sexual behaviour in which HIV could thrive. Many areas of Africa have been particularly hard hit. The epidemic has coincided with drought and famine, civil wars and economic disruption, and the flight of people from the ravaged countryside into cities already overcrowded and impoverished. Cities, historically, have offered newcomers relief from the control and scrutiny of rural conservatism. Where they also offer poverty rather than job opportunities and a new chance in life, prostitution and escapism will ensure that sexual behaviour is not 'safe'. Given also that in many developing countries, the cities provide temporary homes for unattached migrant labourers, both men and women, the passage of HIV between urban and rural communities is assured.

For some time, reports have filtered in of rural areas, especially in Uganda and central Africa, suffering heavy population losses. Like fourteenth-century Europe, whole villages have 'sunk back into the wilderness'. There have been predictions of population implosions wherever the epidemic takes hold. Just how realistic are these dooms-day prophecies? Will a 'third of the world' die? Will AIDS rival that other great twentieth-century killer, the influenza pandemic of 1918–19, which claimed an estimated thirty million lives, the biggest single death toll in history?

The crude exponential growth predictions of the early 1980s have gradually given way to more cautious scenarios. The World Health Organization (WHO) and its Global Programme on AIDS (GPA) which monitor the pandemic, predict that by the year 2000 there will have been between 12 and 18 million AIDS cases, and between 30 and 40 million people will have been infected with HIV worldwide. (*Epidemiological Comments* Vol 20 (11) November 1993:184) In its own authoritative study, *AIDS in the World* (1992), the Global AIDS Policy Coalition predicts figures of up to 110 million infected (p.107) and cumulative AIDS cases of 24 million (p.130). To date, although the highest number of reported AIDS cases is reported from the Americas (371,000 in June 1993), the WHO believes that two-thirds of the estimated 2.5 million cumulative cases have in fact occurred in sub-Saharan Africa.

Reliability of reporting varies, but there is general agreement that the statistics from Africa, and much of the developing world, reflect far fewer AIDS cases than have actually occurred. Poverty, poor health care, inadequate statistics, AIDS-related deaths from the countries' common causes of death, such as tuberculosis (TB) and diarrhoea, and even political manipulation of information, make it difficult to obtain reliable figures.

Not all African countries appear to be equally hit; figures for 1992–93 record 28 cases in Liberia, 13 in Somalia, 31 in Equatorial Guinea. By contrast Uganda had reported 34,000 cases, Malawi 27,000 and Tanzania 39,000 by that period. (*Epidemiological Comments*, Nov.1993:185) (For a comprehensive picture, see *AIDS in the World*:1992)

The new fears are that Asia will feel the next great wave of infections. Although only 3561 Asian cases were reported by June 1993, the WHO believes that over 1.5 million people in South and South-East Asia had been infected by then and that the 'unstable political, social and economic environment in ... Central Asia suggests that the evolution of HIV/AIDS in that part of the world may potentially be rapid' (*Epidemiological Comments:* ibid.:185).

Huge populations are clearly at risk here. In its initial stages the infection rate in communities often doubles in less than a year, and poverty and poor health care accelerate this rate. In affluent First World communities, expensive prophylaxis and treatment for some of the most common opportunistic infections associated with HIV and AIDS are slowly giving AIDS more of the appearance of a chronic, if ultimately fatal, disease. Among the poor everywhere, HIV infection virtually inevitably leads to AIDS and terminal illness within a few years. Whether the pandemic will actually cause populations to shrink is still a matter of hot debate among demographers.

Most Third World countries particularly in sub-Saharan Africa have experienced exponential population growth this century. It seems likely that those experiencing major epidemics will at least experience a slowdown in population growth rates. In a sophisticated demographic modelling exercise, Roy M. Anderson and Robert M. May conclude: 'Available facts indicate that in the absence of major changes in behavior or the development of better drugs, AIDS is likely to cause serious demographic changes in some African countries over the coming decades. It also appears increasingly likely that the pattern will be repeated in parts of India and Southeast Asia.' (1992:25)

When demographers predict slowing or negative population growth as the result of AIDS, they normally attribute this to the failure of 'safer sex' education campaigns to change behaviour. It seems to me that an equally important demographic change could result from successful education programmes that *did* cause major behavioural changes. Many of the births in Africa, for instance, are to young, single mothers in urban areas who, once committed to condom usage to avoid infection, would also avoid these early pregnancies. A successful safer sex message would also presumably mean less extramarital conception in older women. It seems that grassroots understanding of these implications is better than that of some demographers; the whole safer sex message is often dismissed by its recipients as just another attempt to cut back birth rates. Whether people choose to follow the message or not, the results will probably be a slow-down in population growth. Hopefully, this will be due to condoms and fewer partners, rather than the terrible and costly effects of AIDS.

Whatever the ultimate demographic outcome, AIDS will have a very different *modus operandi* from the Black Death or the influenza of 1918-19. Both these pandemics came and went within a short space of time. By the time the first AIDS cases were diagnosed, HIV had already been among us for many years, silently laying the groundwork for an epidemic. The long latency period ensured that the apparently healthy HIV-infected unwittingly spread the virus. Failing a cheap, effective cure or vaccine, HIV could survive in low-level endemic form indefinitely. In the earlier pandemics, most of the millions who were struck down were dead within days. The actual medical cost of each individual illness episode was small; by contrast AIDS, especially among the world's more affluent members, could require years of expensive treatment. In Third World countries, with health budgets already inadequate, even the cost of testing blood for transfusions, could be too much without foreign aid from donors.

The most costly aspect of the AIDS pandemic could be its differential effect on sections of the population. Where the Black Death struck down everyone from newborn babies to old men and women, taking rich and poor, urban and rural alike, HIV is in its primary form a sexually transmitted virus. That haemophiliacs, medical personnel and intravenous drug users exposed to infected blood fall prey, is incidental to its success. The tragic epidemic of paediatric AIDS, among infants born to infected mothers, is also a viral sideshow since its victims will die before they reach sexual maturity. HIV is basically designed to be transmitted by sexually active people. The more sexual activity, the more successful the transmission in any given population. 'Safer sex' – using condoms or limiting the number of partners – will slow it down; multiple partners and an already-high incidence of other sexually transmitted diseases will speed it up.

Its transmission pattern will also skew the population distribution pyramid by selectively removing the very young and those in the age cohort 15 to 55. Because the sexually active and the economically active years tend to coincide, AIDS will have very different effects on the economies of affected societies from the scatter-shot infection of the plague or cholera.

Given the unique circumstances in each society, it is impossible to predict just how economies will be affected or what the global consequences will be. The gay epidemic of the 1980s in America and Europe, for instance, destroyed a significant number of the West's artistic and creative community. The combination of sophisticated medical care and an educated, articulate populace demanding drugs

21

and hospitalization meant each case in the industrialized countries in the 1980s cost between $30,000 and $50,000 per year (Broomberg 1993:39) – a cost comparable to treating other serious illnesses in these countries. As AIDS in the First World becomes increasingly a disease of the poor and marginalized, even the United States' health system has shown the strain. In March 1989, a mayoral panel described the effect on New York as 'not only the city's medical crisis of our times; [it] threatens to become the city's social catastrophe of the century.' With hospitals filled to capacity the health care of all New Yorkers was at risk. (Fox, Aiken and Messikomer 1991:144)

In Third World countries, profiles of the afflicted are still far from clear, but categories such as the military, truck drivers, migrant labourers, urbanites and those involved in commercial sex have been shown to be at risk. Major epidemics among people in these categories would have considerable economic consequences. The military, for instance, are not only trained and maintained at great cost to a country but, weakened by disease, could leave politically or militarily unstable countries subject to upheaval. Mines and urban industries, dependent on skilled and semi-skilled labour would be vulnerable. In Zambia, for instance, the copper mines yield over 90% of the country's export earnings. Comparatively highly trained, the miners would not be easily replaced. Given present trends, 63% of Zambia's skilled labour force could be HIV positive by 2000. (Panos 1992:5) In Zimbabwe, industrialists regard the problem as so serious that they have resorted to the expensive strategy of training two people for each vacancy. (Whiteside and Fitzsimons 1992:18)

Tourism, trade and investment are unlikely to thrive in areas with rampant AIDS epidemics. Even indigenous agriculture would be vulnerable to labour shortages. Women would not only fall ill, but would also be responsible for the care of the ill, both local and those coming home from the cities. As the adults succumbed, children would have to leave school and take over not only the farming, but also the care of the very young and the old. While the personal economic burdens would be intolerably heavy, the epidemic could set back national development by decades. (Panos 1992)

Relative to the industralized countries, actual medical costs will be low, mainly because health care budgets in developing countries are low, and people do not have the personal resources to fund expensive medical care. As the Panos Institute, which has monitored the pandemic since the beginning, points out, the AIDS epidemic hit the developing world at a time of unprecedented economic decline. Foreign debt had risen from $50 billion in 1970 to $1.2 trillion in 1990. In the face of this huge debt and the structural adjustment programs that were implemented in their wake, governments are in the process of cutting back rather than expanding their already over-stretched health systems; the importing of even basic medicines and equipment is often beyond their means. Malnutrition and the resurgence of such old enemies as tuberculosis, malaria, and other sexually transmitted diseases (STDs), especially where they assume drug resistant forms, undermine people's health. STDs, particularly, are associated with increased risks of HIV infection. 'During the 1980s, health spending per capita dropped by over 50% in the poorest 37 countries of Africa and Latin America; in some of these countries, infant mortality has already risen.' (Panos Institute 1992:8) Where the medical cost of an AIDS case in the developed world runs into tens of thousands of dollars, in Zaire the cost will be between $132 and $1585, in Tanzania $104 to $631 and in Zimbabwe an average of $614. (Whiteside and Fitzsimons 1992:13)

It is disconcerting to realize that in such societies, a strongly developed 'funeral culture' – elaborate burial rites with the obligatory involvement and contributions of relatives from local and distant areas – could mean more may be spent on the dead than on the living. It is a hidden cost of the epidemic seldom realized by outsiders.

Such constant reminders of death also take a psychological toll. As Niebuhr wrote, a time of plague 'gnaws the moral stamina and frequently destroys it entirely.' In post-plague medieval Europe, Chaucer's more hedonistic bent notwithstanding, 'themes of youth, exuberance, happiness and joy were played down. The dance of death became a common literary motif. Mystery plays with religious themes also became common, and they usually told of human decay and the torments of hell.' (Gottfried 1983:93) When AIDS first struck the gay communities of the Western World, it arrived at a time of unprecedented cultural activity. The 1960s and 1970s had liberated homosexuals to some extent from the homophobia of the past and their theatre, poetry, novels and music celebrated this new freedom. Within a few years this whole world was to be shattered. For a movement in which sexual freedom, including the freedom to have casual and anonymous sex in the bath-houses and cinemas of cities like San Francisco and New York, had become a symbol of liberation, the recognition that AIDS had changed dramatically the nature of that freedom was to have far-reaching effects. Michael Bronski, active in gay politics for over twenty years, writes of the 'spectre haunting gay life':

It is impossible to be a gay male today and not think of AIDS all the time. Not only are you faced with AIDS every time you read a paper, watch TV, or pick up a magazine ... but AIDS is on your mind every time the telephone rings, every time a letter from a slightly distant friend arrives. (1989:220) ... It has become commonplace over the last five years to assume that a bar regular may be dying or dead if he is absent for a while. Papers, like the *Bay Area Reporter* in San Francisco, run any-

thing from ten to thirty obituaries every week of regular, every-
day men who have died of AIDS. This is a chilling sight,
especially since many people first see the paper in bars and other
gay establishments where it is given away. (1989:221)

Author Andrew Holleran chronicles similar changes in New York
where 'fear now constitutes the substance of homosexual life. AIDS
has been a massive form of aversion therapy. For if you finally equate
sex with death, you don't have to worry about observing safe sex tech-
niques; sex itself will eventually become unappetizing.' (1988:25) –
and, as he remarks wryly: 'Gay life without sex is a theme park.'
(ibid.:68)

How AIDS will affect the psyche of other afflicted communities will
depend not only on the levels of mortality, but also on their expectations of adversity. People who have suffered lives of war, brutality,
famine, poverty and ill-health may simply shrug off AIDS as just
another torment to be endured. (See Chapter 4.)

It is not only gloom, despair and fatalism that greet epidemics.
Although six centuries lie between us and the Black Death, and our
medical understanding of disease has grown greatly in that time,
human behaviour has at root changed little. The fear, anxiety, even
hysteria, which characterized the plague is a pattern which recurs in
virtually all records of epidemics. One exception, despite its ferocity,
was the 1918–19 influenza pandemic, which seemed to evoke a
strangely muted reaction at least in the United States. In his book,
America's Forgotten Pandemic, Alfred Crosby suggests that although
the influenza killed in two months as many Americans as the Germans
had killed in a year, the epidemic which came and went within months,
hit a nation still numbed and preoccupied by the war. The editor of the
New York Times in November 1918 remarked, after 9000 flu deaths in

New York: 'Perhaps the most notable peculiarity of the influenza epidemic is the fact that it has been attended by no traces of panic or even excitement.' (Crosby 1989:313–314) It was indeed a peculiarity. Epidemics throughout history have inspired not only fear and panic, and attempts to flee, but recourse to new religious or magical beliefs aimed at protecting and curing, or even diverting the illness onto someone else. The 'bestial' and 'diabolical' responses to the plague saw the massacre of European Jews and the hysteria of the flagellant movement. The plague of 1656 in Rome saw prostitutes and the poor being marched off to 'pesthouses', and the Jewish ghetto and the poor slum area of Trastevere, where plague had claimed early victims, sealed off and patrolled by guards. 'Violators of public health regulations were fined, summarily executed by firing squads, or hanged from gallows erected in piazzas around the city.' (Risse 1988:39) The cholera pandemics of the nineteenth century, caused by bacteria from human waste polluting water supplies, were seen not as the responsibility of city administrators, but in a classic example of victim-blaming, as the fault of the filth and squalor of the poor who made up the majority of cases. In the New York outbreak of 1832, for instance, harsh measures were sometimes advocated to deal with the slums: 'Turn out the inmates of the place, ventilate and purify the beastly hovels, guard effectively against their return, fence up the streets.' In certain instances compulsory evacuation of the poor to makeshift shanties was actually carried out.' (Risse 1988:45)

In all these instances, the responses did not address the root cause of the epidemic. Like the magical practices described by social anthropologists, they instead served the function of giving people a focus for their fear and an activity to reduce anxiety. Like witch-burning, they sought and found scapegoats.

AIDS, too, produced fear and panic, especially in the early years when its mode of transmission was less fully understood. It came seemingly out of nowhere, confounded medical scientists, who had believed they had infectious diseases pretty much under control, and subjected its victims to a long, and what Susan Sontag calls 'hard' death. The initial epidemic, which rapidly affected tens of thousands of homosexual men, struck at a community already stigmatized. Their 'otherness' was seen by many as the cause of their disease. Later as the disease surfaced among intravenous drug users, black and Latino Americans, and Haitians and Africans, the image of 'otherness' was reinforced; the 'linkage of a horribly frightening disease with stigmatized behaviours and stigmatized groups has characterized the social construction of the epidemic ever since.' (Singer *et al.* 1990:72) In later chapters, the political significance of these linkages will be explored.

Until AIDS, this generation had been spared a major epidemic, and one might have thought that in the last decades of the twentieth century, even if our medical defences proved imperfect, that our social and political responses would have been different, more rational and compassionate, perhaps, then those of earlier times. To examine earlier epidemics is to hold up a mirror to the AIDS generation. We see ourselves again calling for quarantine, isolation, travel restrictions, bans on immigrants, excluding the infected from the use of public schools, swimming pools, hospitals. Rationally, we know that these are pointless exercises. The AIDS virus, we are assured, is not spread by casual contact, and anyway is now so thoroughly dispersed that such measures would do little to contain it.

Yet there is the need to feel protected, to avoid contamination, because AIDS, as Sontag points out, is seen not just as a disease, but as a pollution, a judgement, a divine punishment. (Sontag 1989) That the disease not only manifests itself in stigmatized communities, but produces its own stigmata – lesions, rashes, fungal infestations, physical

27

wasting – serves to deepen the horror and aversion, the irrationality of our responses.

Demands that the authorities 'do something' have, as in previous epidemics, again led to symbolic interventions. The suspension of civil rights such as medical privacy and confidentiality, the harassment of foreign students, especially those of African origin, the tightening up of visa controls to exclude infected – or even 'possibly infected' by virtue of their belonging to 'high risk groups' – visitors, quarantining prostitutes and infected people, are all part of the rusty armoury. Their impotence in the face of AIDS reinforces our pessimism about the ability of authorities, or, for that matter medical and scientific experts, to handle crises of such magnitude. AIDS, like global warming or acid rain, seems to be beyond their scope.

What can governments reasonably be expected to do? It is clear that the control of certain diseases does lie within the direct orbit of state intervention. Typhoid and cholera which can be directly attributed to inadequate sanitation and polluted water require what McNeill would call a 'series of medical and administrative improvements in urban housekeeping.' (1985:254) Other diseases like poliomyelitis, diphtheria or measles respond to programmes of compulsory inoculation, vaccination, or quarantine and treatment. However, until medical science finds a vaccine or cure for AIDS there is in fact no immediate public policy which the state could institute to protect its citizens directly. Much as it might like to do so, it cannot police what happens in the nation's bedrooms. It can only play a role in ensuring that there is funding for research, safe blood supplies and medical procedures, protection of citizens' rights, care for the afflicted and a massive, coordinated effort to ensure that everybody knows the facts of the disease and how to protect themselves against infection.

To carry out these apparently straightforward tasks has proved formidably difficult. Because policy decisions must be made at state level, the AIDS issue is immediately shifted into the political domain. The demands of the healthy, the infected and the ill compete for attention, and their political leverage and status will significantly affect the extent to which their demands will be satisfied. State policy is, however, only the tip of the political iceberg. Decisions surrounding the AIDS issue, such as the allocation of resources, the needs of the healthy and the afflicted, and the protection of individual rights are being made daily in classrooms, doctors' surgeries, insurance offices, on factory floors and political platforms. The outcome of these myriad decisions for individuals, and ultimately for the shape of the AIDS pandemic, will depend on the wider political context in which they are made.

CHAPTER 2

PLAYING WITH FIRE: POLITICIZING AIDS

There is nothing in this whole AIDS mess that is NOT political (Larry Kramer 1990:110 – his emphasis)

L arry Kramer, playwright and fiery campaigner on behalf of the gay community, is probably best known for his attacks on Ronald Reagan ('Hitler' bent on 'gay genocide'), New York's erstwhile mayor Edward Koch and the National Institutes of Health ('murderers' and 'monsters'), but he also constantly sought to goad New York's gays – one million by his calculation – out of their political inaction by his calls to realize the power that lay in their numbers, their wealth and their influence. No matter that the authorities 'intended' their deaths to continue; gay power mobilized could help save them from the epidemic. "Politicians understand only one thing: PRESSURE. You don't apply it – you don't get anything. Simple as that." (1990:174 – his emphasis)

Playing with Fire: politicizing AIDS

Whether any amount of political pressure could turn the epidemic around at this stage is a moot point; what is clear is that those who can make their case heard – those who have access to and control over resources, constituencies and policy-making – will be more likely to benefit from the social and medical palliatives currently available and to influence and benefit from those to come.

When the epidemic struck gay America, they already had considerable political skills, and, as the next chapter describes, the weight of the civil rights culture on their side. They could lobby for anti-discriminatory laws, changes in medical practices, the early release of new drugs, better media coverage, and funding for programmes to care for their ill. They could also mobilize considerable human and financial resources in their own communities from which they drew initially, to set up education programmes, care schemes for the afflicted and political pressure groups to carry out unpopular changes such as closing down the gay bath houses. For a group which only thirty years ago was the target of considerable discrimination, their achievements have been significant.

The American gay organizations' early response to the crisis was repeated in many places around the world. AIDS service organizations (ASOs), driven by 'compassion, fear and anger at indifference' (*AIDS in the World* 1992:775), rapidly formed non-governmental, volunteer-based programmes. In an in-depth survey of these early ASOs in 1992, the Global AIDS Policy Coalition found that in the industrialized countries over half were founded by white, middle-class gay men. In the developing countries they were mostly organized by women, usually with a health, social service or academic background (ibid.:776); they 'shared an immediate challenge to reach beyond their own class, social network, religious affiliation or gender.' (*AIDS in the World* 1992:777) The survey showed the founders of ASOs shared 'a

31

remarkable combination of being somewhat socially marginalized yet politically sophisticated and well connected to sources of financial support within their communities.' (ibid.:778) Since early links with government were usually weak, the ability to raise funds and recruit volunteers was important to the success of these ASOs. Most of them – 70% in industrialized countries and 100% in developing countries – also claimed a broader political agenda than the AIDS issue. Gay or lesbian groups often cited their further liberation or the expansion of universal health care; in developing countries they mentioned expanding public participation in development or support for marginalized groups such as women or commercial sex workers. (ibid.:779)

Initially, the ASOs often worked in isolation from government, either because the AIDS issue was ignored or resisted by the authorities, or because the ASOs wished to retain their autonomy. This separation from, even antagonism to, government programmes, often created a parallel resentment by the ASOs that they were doing the government's job for it. Gay organizations in Europe and America particularly, have felt this; as Tony Whitehead writes of Britain, 'Instead of simply behaving like so many good little Florence Nightingales, developing our own educational and support services within the gay community, we AIDS activists should have fought for such services within the statutory sector.' (1989:107) Such groups, he believes, enabled the government to starve AIDS funding and distance itself from AIDS programmes. A meeting with ASOs and other interested parties, called by the Minister of Health in 1987 for the establishment of the National AIDS Trust to coordinate services and formulate a national strategy, for instance, was not what it seemed. 'The hidden agenda of this meeting was how the government could get away with spending as little as possible. It was quite clear that the Government wanted to get as much money from the community as it possibly could in order to reduce its own level of funding. It was also clear that it wanted to keep itself as far away as possible from any closely targeted education towards gay men and drug users.' (1989:108) Where this kind of suspicion was matched by government or public conviction that gays were making outrageous demands, relative to the AIDS threat or the needs of other health issues, mutual dissatisfaction and recrimination often characterized the AIDS funding debate.

Since 1989, ASOs have not only had increasing direct contact with government, but have also created elaborate ASO networks, which can gain access to AIDS funding, influence the policies and programmes of multilateral organizations such as the WHO and UN, and ensure collective legitimization of policy goals, such as entrenching human rights for HIV/AIDS sufferers. As planned budget cuts in the WHO/ GPA threatened their financing, ASOs also mobilized their networks to try to protect their own continued existence. (*AIDS in the World* 1992:783) The WHO decision to channel funds to ASOs through government programmes after 1992 caused controversy; many ASOs worked with groups such as drug users and prostitutes who might not get support via government funding. (*WorldAIDS* Nov 92:10)

As the epidemic deepens and more ASOs join the established ranks, their continuing role needs careful definition. *AIDS in the World* notes: 'Most ASOs cherish their participation in official consultative bodies, but it is not clear that such participation provides real community input into policy development, as opposed to providing governments and multilateral organizations with the pretence of community consultation while reneging on public responsibilities to respond to the epidemic.' (1992:786)

The problems facing the ASOs exemplify much of the politicking which surrounds AIDS. Forged in the heat of emergency, with dedicated volunteers operating on shoe-string budgets, they dealt with

everything from education programmes, to caring for the sick, to lobbying for changed drug laws. Those who pioneered these movements
talk with nostalgia about the passion and commitment of those early
years – they are 'made to appear more heroic, more fraught with crisis, but withal more closely-knit and unified, than the present, with its
divisive politics.' (Grover 1989:150)

Much of the battle against AIDS has since become routinized and
bureaucratized into what Cindy Patton has branded in the United
States, an 'AIDS industry'. (1989) The growing pandemic necessitat-
ed enormous funding for research, education, prevention, blood safety,
patient care and programme management. By 1990, every country in
the world had established a national AIDS program, though they did
not always conform to WHO standards. (*AIDS in the World* 1992:297)
Funds for these needs come from national sources in industrialized
countries, largely international sources in the developing world. While
most industrial countries, apart from the United States, have national
health care systems that will provide at least some level of health care
(ibid.:315), many developing countries, with health care systems
already in parlous condition, will need international aid to be able to
institute even the most basic programmes, such as education, condom
provision and blood testing. (This will be discussed further in Chapter
4.) After a slow start in 1986 with official development assistance and
international agencies donating $200,000 to developing countries'
AIDS work, funding grew to $255 million in 1990. Since then fund-
ing appears to have been declining, although the pandemic is accelerating in the developing world. (ibid.:511)

Why? Is it a result of economic recession in donor countries? Is it just
'donor fatigue' particularly for Africa? Maureen Law, commenting on
the dwindling sense of urgency in recent years – identified by the
Global Commission on AIDS as one of the critical issues for the 1990s

– suggests that aid has slowed for a number of reasons, such as unrealistic expectations that drugs and vaccines will soon solve the problem, the public perception that the epidemic has levelled off or peaked and is declining in industrialized countries, a growing belief that it is no serious threat to heterosexuals in such countries, and plain weariness with the issues on the part of the public, politicians and the media. Such complacency in wealthy countries may well translate into a failure to increase, or even sustain, funding to those countries experiencing runaway epidemics. (ibid.:322–323)

More alarming is the possibility that if AIDS comes to be seen as a disease of the poor, of the Third World, of 'them' rather than 'us', funders may relegate AIDS to the category of 'just another disease of poverty', like tuberculosis or malaria or leprosy – succumbing to what Cindy Patton calls 'the middle-class view that AIDS is simply a tragic disease, which has been made a political issue by noisy gays and right-wing crazies.' (1989:123) If AIDS demands funding, it will have to do so on the same basis as, and in competition with, other health problems or development needs. It is a possibility Larry Kramer underlined in relation to the gay epidemic in America when he said in a speech in 1987: "The straight world is scared now because they're worried it's going to happen to them. What if it doesn't? Think about that for a while. If all this lethargy is going on now, think what will happen then..." (Kramer 1990:172)

As the pandemic grows and more governmental and non-governmental bodies turn their attention to developing AIDS programmes, in a climate where funding is declining, a battle for scarce resources seems inevitable. In his analysis of shifting patterns in international AIDS financing, Anthony Klouda, coordinator of the AIDS Prevention Unit of the International Planned Parenthood Federation, London, examines the evolution of funding patterns to developing countries, and asks the question: "Who should be funded?" His answer captures the essentially arbitrary, ultimately political, nature of international (and, for that matter, national) funding:

> There have never been any logical criteria in the funding world for choosing one project over another. Mostly, it depends on chance (the particular project has been stumbled on by one representative of the donor), which is then coupled with the current political correctness of the organization seeking funds. When funds are around, there is, of course, competition among organizations for these funds. In these competitions, the most eloquent, the ones with senior officials in high social circles, and the ones with the best knowledge of how to play the game are generally the ones who obtain the bulk of the funds. (*AIDS in the World* 1992:796)

Those fortunate enough to receive funding will often fight to retain their turf and act as 'gatekeepers' to the funding agencies. The politics of funding and patronage can consume such organizations.

By 1991, international AIDS funding for the developing world had amounted to a total of $864 million. (ibid.:512) Although over 80% of current HIV infections occur in developing countries, this amount is a fraction of the AIDS spending in developed countries. For instance, in 1990–91 only about 6% of the total global spending for HIV prevention was in the developing world. North America spent eight times more, and Europe nearly six times more, than the entire developing world. Per capita, North America spent $2.71, Europe $1.18, sub-Saharan Africa $0.07 and Latin America $0.03 on prevention. AIDS care costs were similarly disproportionately spent in industrialized countries. (ibid.:5–6)

Funding for research projects is almost entirely confined to the industrialized countries, where a cumulative amount of approximately $5.45
billion had been spent by the end of 1991. United States spending
alone rose from $4 million in 1982 to $1.28 billion in 1991. (ibid.:261)
Like funding for developing countries' AIDS programmes, AIDS
research funding also appears to have reached a plateau. Along with
the pandemic, funds grew by leaps and bounds between 1985 and
1991. In 1991, funding grew by just 10%, barely ahead of inflation let
alone the pandemic's wildfire spread (ibid.:263). Again we need to ask
the question whether this slowdown reflects the economic recession or
the fact that the industrialized countries no longer feel threatened by
the epidemic. As the global dynamic is lost, there is a danger that
AIDS programmes, whether they be research, prevention or care ori-
entated could degenerate into *ad hoc* local and national responses, driven by pressure groups rather than the real needs of any particular
community.

Nevertheless, an AIDS breakthrough is obviously Nobel Prize territory. There has been feverish, indeed unseemly, competition among
scientists at major institutions, particularly in the United States and
Europe to make that breakthrough. The bitter controversy between
two highly respected researchers, Robert Gallo of the National
Institutes of Health (NIH) in Bethesda, Maryland and Luc Montagnier
of the Pasteur Institute in Paris, is symptomatic of the heat this struggle has generated. Both men isolated and identified a virus, later to
become known as HIV, which they believed could be the cause of
AIDS; both published their preliminary findings in the May 1983 issue
of *Science* (Gallo 1991:151). The Gallo laboratories then went on to
develop a blood test for antibodies to the virus, known as Elisa –
Enzyme Linked Immunosorbent Assay – which could determine
whether an individual had been exposed to the virus. An acrimonious
battle followed centering on whether the viral material on which the

37

Gallo laboratories based its research had been contaminated with material that actually originated in Montagnier's laboratory. It culminated in litigation, with the French challenging the US government's patent on the Elisa test, Gallo finally acknowledging that the Montagnier virus had contaminated the American material, and his being hauled before a US government panel on charges of scientific misconduct.

It was a sorry end to a process that had started out as a co-operative scientific quest. Although Gallo's laboratory remains in the forefront of AIDS research, much energy was wasted by the scandal. "I'll wonder all my life what else we could have done if we hadn't been interrupted for seven or eight years, five years heavy duty," Gallo said in a *Newsweek* interview. (August 23, 1993:54) His colleagues, too, fear the negative effect this has had on the scientific process. One commented: 'The message to young government scientists is that you will operate in an environment where there is no distinction between error and fraud and where you are subjected to the whims of the political process.' (ibid.:55) In 1994, the US Congress undertook a massive overhaul of its AIDS research funding. Proposed by AIDS activists and supported by some scientists, it aimed to co-ordinate research spending under a strengthened Office of AIDS Research at the NIH; the aim was to eliminate research duplication at the many different NIH institutes, described by their critics as 'fiefdoms'. (*WorldAIDS* May 1993:4)

Researchers in other fields fume that the extravagant search for AIDS' Holy Grail is happening at their expense, and indeed is costing lives that their research or even existing medical interventions, could easily save from the virus. Chief critics are people working in the field of sexually transmitted diseases. It has been established beyond any doubt that STDs, particularly those which cause lesions through which

HIV can easily enter the bloodstream, are a major AIDS risk factor. Although there has been some improvement, STDs remain a poor relation in the funding stakes. (See *AIDS in the World* 1992:301–304 for discussion.) In 1993, funding for STDs in the US federal budget was $103 million, for AIDS research $1.3 billion. A *Newsweek* report comments acidly:

> That huge commitment reflects both the political savvy of the gay community and America's enduring faith in technological fixes. State of the art laboratories, full of brilliant scientists racing to understand a deadly medical mystery, have a lot more popular appeal than storefront clinics in bombed-out neighbourhoods. Both have their place. But storefront clinics have the advantage of being able to combat AIDS today. (June 21, 1993:49)

With the AIDS stakes so high it is not surprising that individuals, laboratories, even governments, should be willing to throw themselves into the fray. Nor is it surprising that AIDS projects remain under the international spotlight. This spotlight will, for instance, be focused on the whole tricky process of vaccine testing. Who will be the guinea pigs? Will scientists pick those wealthy First Worlders considered to be at special risk, or Third Worlders where galloping epidemics are ravaging whole countries? Either way, bystanders could cry "foul", accusing First Worlders of undue influence or those opting for Third World trials of using the poor as research fodder. There has already been much criticism of the 'quick and dirty' methods of AIDS researchers who invade a community, do hasty research, leave, and write a paper for a journal or conference; the host community never sees the results or any benefit from their 'participation'. Even if a vaccine were found, some doubt whether it would ever help developing countries too poor to pay.

Research decisions are very much at the mercy of the vagaries of the political process. Vaccine research in Rwanda was a case in point, as Claude Raynaut of the University of Bordeaux discovered. In April 1993, the Rwandan Ministry of Health in cooperation with the WHO, organized a workshop in the capital, Kigali, to clarify the planned vaccine trials. Given that Rwanda was already suffering a heavy AIDS burden – 1101 AIDS cases per million population in November 1992 – their eligibility for urgent intervention was not in question. The news of the trial led to high expectations and a stream of volunteers wishing to participate. Such trials always raise complex medical and ethical issues, for instance obtaining informed consent, or using control groups who would be given placebos – neutral and harmless vaccine substitutes – rather than the potentially useful drug. In Rwanda's case, testing raised equally complex political issues. Raynaut commented:

It is not inconceivable that in the context of the country's troubled political climate, such trials will become an important issue for opposing political, ideological and religious forces. We cannot simply avoid this matter, by protesting that it is political rather than scientific or technical. The very feasibility of the trials themselves may well depend on the response to this question. *(Sociétés d'Afrique & SIDA* No. 2 Oct 1993:2–3)

As it turned out, it was the country's 'troubled political climate', culminating in the Rwandan massacres of 1994, which put paid to the vaccine trials. With more than half a million Rwandans dead and millions having fled to refugee camps in Tanzania and Zaire, AIDS dropped far down on the country's list of priorities. War and upheaval are great allies of the AIDS pandemic, as Chapter 4 will show.

Rwanda provides an extreme case of politics defeating people's AIDS efforts, but, at a time where the only real strategies we have to contain the pandemic depend on sex education and behavioural change, any political, ideological or religious grouping that stands to lose from an AIDS campaign – or benefit from opposing it – may elect to pursue its own goals rather than do battle with the virus. Since the control of information can become a life or death matter, who is reached or not reached, may also be a political consideration. Are those at risk part of your constituency? If so, taking a strong line on AIDS programmes may be politically expedient; if not, ignoring the issue, or even fighting against programmes, may increase your popularity. Are those at risk a minority without political clout? Ignoring, blaming or stigmatizing them cannot do you much harm, and may even earn you support. Perhaps you believe that withholding information from the country's population or the international community is to your political or economic advantage? Perhaps tourism and investment could be influenced by declaring an epidemic? Initial denial, even concealment by the government in Zimbabwe, for instance, meant that in 1987 the Ministry of Health actually reduced the number of cases reported to date. People with AIDS were officially discouraged from making their illness public; at one point a ministry spokesman even accused the medical profession of misdiagnosis and over-reporting. The new health minister, Dr Timothy Stamps, insisted that the country be given the true facts, but the delay had cost valuable time. (Whiteside 1993:218–219) (Some of the complex issues determining African states' reactions to the AIDS issue are discussed in Chapter 3.)

Because AIDS often disproportionately affects marginalized or stigmatized groups, and concerns issues like sex, disease and death, which are everywhere hedged around with complex cultural values and taboos, any AIDS programme is vulnerable to ideological manipulation. Sometimes this involves the purely political manoeuvres discussed above; at other times, it reflects deeper social values which are

41

contradicted by the pragmatic demands of AIDS prevention and care. For instance, at the first Sino-American AIDS meeting in Beijing in November 1990, Chinese delegates not only denounced sex outside marriage, but also affirmed their faith in 'propaganda' as a mechanism for dealing with the epidemic.

> Wrong behaviour which violates the biological and sociological laws has to incur the double punishment of nature and society .... The wild spread of AIDS is the most severe penalization .... In China, health education for the prevention of AIDS never includes the use of condoms, and our guiding principle is mainly ... [to warn] against non-marital sexual relations and [to advocate] sexual morality. (Zhu quoted in Gil 1994:18)

Elsewhere, the need for gay education, for instance, can run counter to existing legislation which still regards homosexual activity as a criminal offence. The common belief that children should be spared 'the facts of life', lest they corrupt young minds and bodies, can make AIDS education in schools impossible – even in societies where teenage pregnancy and STDs bear ample witness to ignorance being no guarantee of innocence. Condoms for prisoners and prostitutes, clean needle exchanges for drug addicts, AIDS programmes for the mentally retarded – many strategies involve uncomfortable compromises with issues to which we would rather turn a blind eye. (One small benefit we might derive from AIDS, is that we will be forced to drop some of the hypocrisies of our social policies in order to confront this pandemic.)

Perhaps one of the most vexed issues of all is the conflict between deeply held religious beliefs and AIDS prevention in countries with powerful religious leaders. While fundamentalist religious sects everywhere have raised issues around AIDS as a punishment for sin,

exacerbating homophobia, racism and xenophobia, the more significant problems stem from mainstream religious influence on the imple-
mentation of AIDS prevention campaigns. The most powerful pres-
sures have come from Muslim and Roman Catholic leaders.

In Islamic countries this has ranged from flatly denying that AIDS
could become a problem in a devout Muslim community, to providing
half-hearted information, stopping short of even mentioning condoms.

At a landmark conference on 'The role of religion and moral behaviour
in the Prevention and Control of AIDS and STDs', held in Cairo in
September 1991, leading Muslim and Coptic Christian theologians
'rejected safer sex education and condoms and affirmed that early marriage and marital faithfulness are more appropriate weapons against
HIV infection.' (*WorldAIDS* March 1992:3)

It is an attitude that causes many observers concern. Self-congratula-
tory analyses based on the morality and virtue of your followers can
rapidly turn sour as modern realities sweep away conservative values.
In Egypt itself, where it was an accepted tradition for young men to
frequent prostitutes before marriage, there is growing concern that the
annual influx of two million tourists will provide a conduit between the
pandemic and the Egyptian people. (ibid.) Already sex tourism to
Muslim countries such as Algeria, Morocco and Tunisia has been
implicated in HIV transmission. Tourism is a major foreign exchange
earner and medical officers in Morocco and Tunisia have accused their
governments of 'bowing to pressure from the travel industry and
silencing reports on the spread of the virus.' (*WorldAIDS* March
1992:6)

Some Muslim countries have tried to balance the religious sensibilities
of their people against the urgent needs for AIDS prevention. Yemen,

for instance, realizing that the tens of thousands of migrant workers who commute to neighbouring states were potentially at risk of exposure, acted even before there was any evidence of an epidemic. The campaign is addressed particularly to those who travel abroad, but government leaflets 'stop short of advising on 'safe sex' with condoms in recognition of Islamic opposition to sex outside of marriage.' (*WorldAIDS* March 1992:3) Whether Islamic countries will deny their risk, believing that AIDS is a disease of the immoral West, implement Islam-based campaigns (as has happened with some success in northern Nigeria), wage limited campaigns (like Yemen), condemn immorality, but tacitly allow programmes (as Indonesia has done), or go for a pragmatic strategy stripped of moral content, will very much depend on the changing balance of popular conservatism, the relative power of political and religious leaders and the depredations of the epidemic.

The same factors influence Christian, particularly Roman Catholic, communities. From Catholic areas as widespread as Latin America, the Philippines, Kenya and Papua New Guinea come reports of the agonizing choices Catholic leaders and their congregations face.

The growing epidemics are already evidence of the flouting of church teaching that sex is an activity allowed only within the confines of Holy matrimony; to recommend the use of condoms would not only seem to condone this behaviour, but to undermine the Church's passionately held stand on birth control. Because they are a contraceptive, the Vatican refuses to condone the use of condoms under any circumstances. In many places the influence of the Church has succeeded in preventing state programmes, and closing down those started by other organizations. In Mexico, MEXFAM, the Mexican Family Planning Association, affiliated to the International Planned Parenthood Federation, faced a 'well-orchestrated' pro-lifers' campaign against its

44

sex information, films, videos and booklets; 'its professed intention was to put pressure on the government in order to obtain MEXFAM's closure,' a campaign which had some local success, but failed nationally as MEXFAM picked up official support. (Juárez 1993:33) In Peru, the Health Ministry, pressured by conservative sectors of the population including the Association of Catholic Doctors, blocked condom commercials on television; the conservatives argued that AIDS prevention programmes were not necessary for people with morals. (*WorldAIDS* March 1993:10) In Papua New Guinea, where the number of HIV infections is still small, very high rates of STDs are an ominous pointer to things to come. A highly successful social marketing programme of coloured condoms in urban areas, was almost derailed by the national censorship board, because the packaged instruction inserts were deemed pornographic, and distributors were ordered to remove them. In a compromise settlement, the line drawings were modified. Church opposition to condoms is very strong. Despite a statement by a Catholic church medical liaison committee representative that condom use for disease prevention would be sanctioned, 'Catholic nursing sisters and others in mission-run health centres are resisting their promotion and distribution. One group made a poster showing that the natural holes in latex condoms were larger than the size of a single virus (which is not the case), effectively discouraging condom usage.' Elsewhere missionaries have managed to pressure pharmacies into moving condoms from the open shelves to under the counter. (*WorldAIDS* Sept 1993:1–2)

Brazil has followed much the same policy pattern as other Catholic countries, where educational campaigns have been revised 'not to increase their effectiveness, but to avoid offending moral sensibilities,' (Daniel and Parker 1993:24) although, given a considerable liberal/ left faction in the Church, there has been regional policy variation. Strong pressure from the Church has, for instance, meant that all reference to condoms has at times been eliminated from government-sponsored advertisements. (ibid.:119) With a growing epidemic, increasingly moving into the heterosexual community, the church position seems anachronistic. Nothing underlines this more strongly than the appearance of the disease among its own priests. *WorldAIDS* reports that in São Paulo, for instance, 25 priests are believed to have died of AIDS between 1989 and 1994. Although accurate statistics on such a taboo subject are obviously difficult to find, the report quotes a senior source in the Church suggesting that more than 40 priests could be seriously ill. (*WorldAIDS* Sept 1994:11) Indications of modes of transmission are even more elusive. To insist, as some have, that it is a result of caring for AIDS patients, would only serve to mystify the issue further, and confound attempts to equip Brazilians with the facts. It could also serve to erode the Church's influence on the government, which some believe has happened since the 1980s. An AIDS programme official notes, for instance, that the vague 'AIDS kills' message of the 1980s, has been replaced by government pamphlets carrying step-by-step illustrated instructions on condom use. In the 1980s, any campaign which even mentioned condoms was vetoed by the Church. (ibid.)

The issue of religious interventions on the AIDS front is far from simple. Secular organizations, both to reinforce their own claims on funding and constituencies, and out of frustration at the moralism and conservatism of religious alternatives, often fail to appreciate the importance of such inputs. Long before today's ASOs, religious workers often offered poor people their only access to medical care and health education. In places where religious beliefs provide the core values which influence people's behaviour, the message of chastity and monogamy can undoubtedly be a powerful protection. It may be imperfect, but the increasingly depressing news about the limited, often negligible, effect of AIDS information on actual behaviour, particularly condom use, suggests that AIDS workers cannot afford to be dismissive of any help they can get. More importantly, perhaps, among those who will suffer and die in the pandemic, particularly in the developing world, compassionate religious care and solace may be all there is on offer.

A danger in church programmes is that while they may provide care and encourage a safer lifestyle, they may simultaneously use the infected as object lessons on the consequences of a fall from moral grace. Such preaching not only adds to the anguish of the afflicted; it also increases the tendency to stigmatize AIDS sufferers, and often also their families. The misery, for instance, which Kenya's Anglican minister Reverend Stephen Njenga creates by refusing to bury AIDS cases – he would rather have one follower than 'a thousand who indulge in immoral practices' (*WorldAIDS* Nov 1993:12) – must be offset against the good the Church can do. It faces particularly thorny problems in working with people like prostitutes and street kids, where failure to provide safer sex information amounts to ignoring their needs. Peter Dalglish of Street Kids International, a Canada-based voluntary organization, says:

> We are concerned that the religious agenda can affect the way the organization responds to the needs of kids. Most religious organizations are very reluctant to talk about sexuality, sexual abuse, sexual identity, HIV transmission, safe sex, contraception, masturbation and issues considered to be 'women's issues' – all of which concern street kids directly. (*WorldAIDS* Jan 1994:9)

Conservatism, of course, is not limited to religious conservatism. Squeamishness about public discussion of sexual issues is found around the globe; the idea that ignorance is innocence is one of humanity's commoner myths. Government information packages may face resistance at community level; enough local pressure may add up to a veto on central campaigns. The younger the audience targeted, and the more explicit the information, particularly regarding condoms, the more likely there is to be public resistance. Faced with this, it is easy to see why conservative countries have chosen to focus on issues like blood transmission, or the role of foreign visitors and migrants, or prostitutes, rather than alienate political constituencies.

Unfortunately, AIDS is a relentless foe. Unless it is met unblinkingly, head-on, people will not be able to face it down. At present our only major weapons, apart from medical palliatives, are strategies for behavioural change. 'Safer sex' depends on both personal restraint and condom usage. ASOs, NGOs, governments and religious leaders will all eventually have to acknowledge this. To date, their competing agendas have often produced garbled messages and an indecorous squabbling over constituencies, policies and resources. In fundamental ways, we have failed to mobilize effectively against a common threat. We cannot afford to face the next decade in such disarray. There is a need for concerted action. As Tom Stoddard writes:

> AIDS is unlike any other public health issue. In each individual and in the body politic, it spurs sentiments that are likely to interfere with rational resolution of the crisis. AIDS requires special political leaders who will put public health concerns first, who will not shy from controversy, and who will step forward to mould and inform public opinion. (1989:106)

It remains to be seen whether such leaders will emerge, or whether they can control the hydra-headed politics of this epidemic.

My own country, South Africa, provides an object lesson of just how tightly an AIDS crisis can be woven into the whole political web. (For a fuller account, see van der Vliet 1994.) South Africa currently has close to two million infected people in a population of 43 million. The initial epidemic in the predominantly white, middle-class homosexual community receded in the face of concerted gay 'safer sex' campaigns, but, since 1987, a heterosexual epidemic in the predominantly black (African) community has been gathering pace, with infection rates currently doubling every 15 months. Spared an injecting drug problem, the new epidemic has been almost entirely fuelled by heterosexual transmission, between people with no other major risk factors. Black communities make up 76% of South Africa's population, with 37% under 15 years of age, a figure which will rise to 50% by 2000. (*SAIRR Survey* 1993/94:48)

The disastrous potential of such an epidemic – economically, socially and psychologically – should have triggered massive, concerted action to inform the public and plan for consequences. Many organizations including gay associations, some local authorities, clinics, businesses, trade unions, and church, welfare and civic associations did respond with invaluable prevention and care projects. As elsewhere, their efforts were often hampered by lack of resources and coordination, and a population and its leaders apparently unmotivated by any sense of national urgency.

At least part of the explanation for this is that, since the beginning, the AIDS issue has been heavily politicized. This is not a uniquely South African problem, but as Refiloe Serote of the Township AIDS Programme observes, "the political and racial divisions, created and inflamed by apartheid, make everything to do with AIDS 'political'." (*WorldAIDS* Nov 1990:5)

Under the previous government, a tiny AIDS budget, inappropriate programmes, insufficient consultation and puritanical attitudes to sex education in black and white communities crippled information initiatives. The universal problems of disbelief and denial were aggravated by distrust and suspicion of government campaigns in the black community. Where were all these sick people? Were condoms and fewer partners just new weapons in the government's 'genocidal' population programme? If people believed in AIDS at all, they speculated about its origins. Had it been fabricated in an 'imperialist' laboratory, or was it being sprayed on crowds in police tear-gas attacks? Were infected haemophiliacs or infected ex-ANC guerillas being used to spread the disease in black communities? (van der Vliet 1994) As AIDS activist and long-time apartheid opponent, Dr Ivan Toms observed of the old regime, there was "no possibility that the government could, even if it [had] the inclination, run an effective campaign to limit the spread of HIV infection. It [has] no credibility, or legitimacy whatsoever among blacks." (Toms 1990:14)

For their part, right-wing politicians used the threat of an epidemic in the black community to stir up racial prejudice, win political support and demand renewed segregation, by suggesting that AIDS could be passed on in social or physical contact in desegregated facilities such as schools, hospitals and swimming pools. Oblivious of its human and economic costs, many believed it could 'solve' the country's political and demographic problems. Conservative Party member of parliament Clive Derby-Lewis (later imprisoned for his role in the assassination of black political leader Chris Hani) was quoted as saying "If AIDS stops black population growth, it would be like Father Christmas." (van der Vliet 1994:113–114)

The April 1994 elections and the transition to democracy were necessary steps to a more credible AIDS policy. Nevertheless, AIDS will now have to compete for human and financial resources with all the country's other urgent needs, such as housing, education, jobs, health care, basic infrastructure. Whether an as-yet silent epidemic will be seen as a priority is far from clear.

AIDS and the safer sex message is unpopular as a political platform in most places. To bring this message to a community where research has repeatedly shown condoms to be unpopular, and particularly to the militant young, who have just emerged from more than a decade of brutality, violence and disruption in their communities, is politically risky.

Some, especially in the trade unions, have tried to make the message more palatable by coating it in a political sweetener – suggesting that AIDS is a disease of apartheid and the impoverished conditions it created, and will yield to a political solution. While social regeneration will help to turn the tide (see Chapter 4), it is not a short-term strategy. Such arguments need to be balanced by a very strong message that the only immediate solution to the problem is behavioural change. To take such a stance requires political courage. As Stoddard says, it requires special political leaders to ignore the controversy and prioritize public health issues. (1989:106) In President Nelson Mandela, South Africa has such a leader. He has repeatedly broached the subject on public platforms and pleaded for the issue to be depoliticized; the issue, he said, did not allow anyone "the luxury of political bias or hearts-and-minds winning exercises." (*The Argus* 23 October 1992) Whether his message will be heard above the din of politics remains to be seen.

CHAPTER 3

STIGMATIZED VICTIMS: RISK, BLAME AND DISCRIMINATION

Many illnesses transform their victims into a stigma-tized class, but AIDS is the first epidemic to take stig-matized classes and make them victims.
Richard Goldstein (1989:84)

The history of a disease is often paralleled by a history of inhu-manity to its sufferers. Sometimes sufferers become social outcasts, like the leper in Leviticus, forced to wear torn clothes, to warn off others with the cry "unclean, unclean", and to 'dwell alone in a habitation outside the camp' (Chapter 13:45–46), or the yellow fever victim in nineteenth-century America who would be left to die alone, or thrown out 'to seek asylum in a public hospital, to avoid dying in the street.' (Musto 1988:73) Sometimes, too, old pre-judices pin epidemics on readymade conventional scapegoats; blaming medieval Jews for the plague or New York's Irish immigrants for the nineteenth century cholera epidemic are cases in point.

52

AIDS, as Goldstein notes, is unique in that those who were actually afflicted were already victims of prejudice and discrimination. No social manipulation of facts was necessary; the disease struck directly at groups who were already marginal. Its initial targets were homosexuals and Africans, followed shortly by drug users and the poor and wretched in their myriad forms. They were people who had rejected, or been rejected by, what was seen as mainstream America and Europe. Writing of Brazil, Herbert Daniel and Richard Parker comment: 'Prostitutes, prisoners, transvestites, street children and drug addicts, for example, have all taken their place alongside homosexuals within the imagery conjured up by the mention of AIDS, and have become part of an ever-expanding vision not only of marginality, but, by extension, of danger.' (Daniel and Parker 1993:53) The coincidence of a new disease, in marginalized communities, in troubled and insecure times was a recipe for a new wave of prejudice.

Believing that AIDS affected 'them' not 'us' meant people could deny they were at risk. By associating HIV with 'risk groups', rather than risky behaviour, even the proverbial sailor with a girl in every port could believe he was safe – as long as he was not gay, black or injecting drugs. China denied it was at risk because AIDS was a disease of the decadent West (*WorldAIDS* Jan 1993:14); Romania's Ceaucescu dismissed it as 'a capitalist disease'. (*WorldAIDS* Nov 1990:2) Middle Eastern Muslim leaders believed that their religion would protect them. (*WorldAIDS* March 1992:3) In Britain, despite extensive public education campaigns, a report quotes Asian immigrants saying that AIDS was a disease of bored white Britons, who went in for sexual experimentation; some even believed that Asians were biologically immune to AIDS. (*The Guardian* 15-04-1992) Other Britons may be just as sceptical; teenagers in Norfolk told researchers that they thought the media were exaggerating, "shoving some figures down your throat – so they can stop you having sex." (*WorldAIDS* March

1991:7–8) Where whole communities or countries adopt such stances, it becomes difficult to raise AIDS awareness, because denial has been invested with elements of parochial superiority.

While some conspiracy theorists believe AIDS is a myth, others believe the epidemic is actually far worse than the authorities admit, and that they are deliberately concealing information for political purposes. So Dr David Seftel can accuse the South African government of allowing uncounselled infected black haemophiliacs to spread the disease into the community: "The regime is generating genocide." (1988:21) (There have been three black cases of haemophiliac transmission to date – an unlikely basis for a genocidal programme.) Outspoken AIDS activist, Larry Kramer, repeatedly accused Ronald Reagan's administration of similar murderous intentions: "There's only one word to describe his monumental disdain for the dead and dying: genocide." (Kramer 1990:158) In Haiti, at the time of the collapse of the hated Duvalier regime in 1986, some people speculated about whether the Duvaliers had actually caused AIDS. Others felt that though the Duvaliers had been able to create zombies, they were too stupid to create AIDS – although they had possibly allowed their nation to be used as guinea pigs by the Americans in a plan to stem migration. (Farmer 1990:13)

The idea that AIDS has been deliberately manufactured for political purposes, to eliminate either an enemy or a marginalized group, surfaces regularly. In one study in the United States, for instance, 35% of 1056 black church members in five cities believed that AIDS is a form of genocide, while 30% remained unsure. A story circulating in Uganda accuses the United States of distributing AIDS-infected condoms in Africa. In the former Soviet Union, AIDS was said to have been developed from a lentiretrovirus found in sheep, as part of a US military programme on germ warfare. AIDS researcher Robert Gallo;

commenting on this theory, writes: 'The notion was simply stupid, malicious or both. Still some people seem capable of believing any nonsense, so long as it reinforces their prejudices or supports their politics.' (Gallo 1991:220)

AIDS has proved a fertile field for both prejudice and politics, dangerously politicizing AIDS in a revival of racism and homophobia. The fact that the first victims were from stigmatized groups unleashed a wave of victim blaming. For those who had experienced the 1960s and 1970s as a threatening floodtide of change, overwhelming their countries with a sexual revolution that liberated women and homosexuals, racial desegregation, a huge influx of immigrants and a culture of drugs, violence and crime, the AIDS epidemic symbolized divine retribution. That it struck first at gays and injecting drug users, made it seem like a prophecy fulfilled. It not only punished the 'guilty', but appeared to reward the 'blameless' and set to rights the balance which they felt had tipped against them. Even for those who saw no element of the divine in the disease, or perhaps saw it as 'nature striking back', there was a feeling that the victims deserved their fate; it was their own fault.

What of those infected who could not be shown to deserve it? Some sufferers, especially in the days before the nature of the virus was understood, were infected by blood transfusions, or, in the case of haemophiliacs, by blood products. They, and the growing number of babies infected *in utero* or during breast-feeding by HIV positive mothers, came to be called the 'innocent victims' – implying of course, that the others were guilty. It was the ability of the 'guilty' to spread the disease to the 'innocent' – to wives, to babies and others who did not fit the risk-group categories – that made AIDS a useful weapon in the hands of religious fundamentalists and political demagogues. The interlinking of three of humankind's most potent emotional themes –

55

sex, disease and death – made for riveting oratory. By stirring up fear against groups and then offering solutions, bigots have always rein- forced prejudices and strengthened their own constituencies. In November 1984, for instance, two weeks before a federal parliamen- tary election in Australia, the Queensland government reported that three babies had died of AIDS-related illnesses after being given blood from an HIV-infected donor. In the public hysteria that followed, the federal leader of the right-wing National Party declared that "If it wasn't for the promotion of homosexuality as a norm by Labor, I am quite confident that the deaths of these poor babies would not have occurred." (*WorldAIDS* March 1991:10)

In Western Europe, growing fear of economic immigrants, and politi- cal asylum seekers following the dissolution of the Eastern bloc, has led to increasing stigmatization and violence against those labelled risk groups, particularly in the growing European ultra-right movements. In France, for instance, Jean-Marie le Pen's racist campaigns exploit- ed fears by demanding mandatory nationwide testing and quarantine for all those found to be infected. (Sontag 1989:62) A poster for Le Pen's *Front National* which polled 18.9% in regional French elections in 1992, proclaimed: 'AIDS equals socialism, immigration, drugs and political racketeering.' (*WorldAIDS* July 1992:10) Muslim fundamen- talists in Malaysia have urged the execution of homosexuals and pros- titutes as a way of preventing the epidemic. (*WorldAIDS* Nov 1991:6) Latin American paramilitary death squads are reported as 'continuing to harass and murder gays across the continent in the wake of the AIDS epidemic.' (ibid.:5)

Another variant on the political theme insists that 'decent folk' are not at risk, and denounces the 'hysteria' surrounding AIDS. In the United States, protagonists of this viewpoint believe that 'the excessive pub- licity given the disease' stems from 'the desire to placate an all-pow-

erful minority by agreeing to regard 'their' disease as 'ours' – further
evidence of the sway of nefarious 'liberal' values and of America's
spiritual decline.' (Sontag 1989:64–65) Policy decisions outlawing
discrimination against people with AIDS, prompted conservative
columnist Patrick Buchanan to protest. 'Has America become a country where classroom discussion of the Ten Commandments is imper-
missible but teacher instructions in safe sodomy are to be mandatory?'
(Quoted in Sontag 1989:65) Unfortunately, the fear of being tainted by
association with such reactionary views, may well prevent national
debate of alternative views of the AIDS issue.

How successful this exploitation of AIDS and its association with stigmatized groups is in attracting or retaining the support of a constituency, is uncertain. What is certain is that it has caused fear and anger
among those it targets, driven them underground where they become
harder to reach with AIDS programmes, and politicized the issue of
AIDS in ways that make rational policies and programmes more difficult to implement.

The so-called African epidemic well illustrates what happens when
politics and old prejudices meet in an epidemic.

To talk of an 'African epidemic' is itself problematic. Demographic
information and HIV/AIDS statistics are often incomplete, but it seems
clear that even if we exclude North Africa, where incidence appears to
be low, sub-Saharan Africa shows very variable infection rates. WHO
figures for 1992, for instance, show that while Malawi had 2563 AIDS
cases per million people, Uganda 1841, Zimbabwe 1290, Tanzania
1268 and Kenya 1190, many countries registered a hundred or less per
million. Some of these statistics are patently too low, since monitoring
HIV levels in seroprevalence surveys on, for instance, blood donors or
ante-natal testing, reveals higher rates. While African infection rates

vary greatly, some of the worst hit areas show HIV rates of 20% and more among the sexually active population, especially in the urban areas. (*WorldAIDS* May 1993:6–7) Nevertheless, there are places like the Gambia, Chad, Cameroon, Lesotho, Guinea and Namibia where the levels were still well under 2% HIV infected in 1992. (ibid.) Many writers believe that 2% represents the infection level at which the epidemic begins to spiral out of control.

Sensationalist writers and commentators ignored the finer points; decades of the Biafran war, the Congo bloodshed, and war and famine in Somalia and Ethiopia had primed their readers to expect large scale catastrophes from the Dark Continent. Headlines like 'Africa's New Agony', 'Nightmare of a Raddled City' and 'Sickening of a Continent' followed the pattern. They were seized on by Africans as blatant lies, reinforcing racist views of the continent and making Africa 'the poor scapegoat of AIDS'. (Chirimuuta and Chirimuuta 1987:Chapter 9) Sadly, developments since the Chirimuuta book was published have revealed that there are areas of Africa that have suffered terribly as the epidemic grew, but the early sensational media response must take some of the responsibility. Africans and their governments often responded to this perceived racism by retreating into denial and blame. There were bitter repudiations and counter-accusations – that, for instance, the WHO had introduced HIV in its vaccination programmes, or that AIDS was a fabrication of the West to bring down birth rates in Africa through condom use, or that the virus had been manufactured in imperialist laboratories. By refusing to admit the extent of the problem, or to begin informing and educating the populace, valuable time was lost.

The suggestion that the virus might have originated in Africa caused a storm of protests. Scientists, probably without even considering that there might be such an emotional reaction, speculated that the virus might have ancient, and possibly relatively benign roots in Africa, but that circumstances such as social upheaval, urbanization, poor health or some factor as yet unknown had changed its nature. Recent research by, for instance, evolutionary biologist, Paul Ewald, appears to support this theory. If it proves to be true, it could provide valuable information on the nature of the virus, on how it becomes lethal and how it could be tamed. Such scientific speculation was not, as Cindy Patton suggests, because the scientists believed 'nothing of this sort could have arisen in the germ-free West.' (Patton 1990:83) Scientists were well aware of the many infectious diseases such as measles, mumps, diphtheria and smallpox, which Europeans had carried to other lands. More recently, in 1976, the outbreak of Legionnaire's disease in Philadelphia at a meeting of members of the American Legion, showed new – or apparently new – epidemic diseases could originate anywhere. In this instance, it was traced to an airborne bacterium, named *Legionella*, thriving in the air-conditioning system, perhaps an instance of an old bacterium flourishing due to new technology. (Gallo 1991:131)

Those who protested against the African origin hypothesis believed that AIDS was being blamed on Africa, that Africa was somehow being held responsible for the epidemic. They believed, too, that it was just another example of the world's profoundly racist views of the continent. The Chirimuutas write that 'the association of black people with dirt, disease, ignorance and an animal-like sexual promiscuity' made it 'almost inevitable that black people would be associated with [AIDS'] origin and transmission.' (Chirimuuta and Chirimuuta 1987:1) Sexually transmitted diseases are invariably stigmatized, and blamed on the 'other'; in 1495, for instance, the first recorded syphilis epidemic was initially labelled the 'French disease' by the Italians, and the 'Neapolitan disease' by the French; in time both agreed to call it the Spanish disease. (Gallo 1991:129) Given the long history of racism, the hypersensitivity of Africa to being associated with AIDS is understandable, but dangerous. In Nigeria, for instance, where by the end of 1992, over half a million people were believed to be infected, many Nigerians still scoff at the idea of an epidemic. 'Cynics call AIDS 'the white man's disease'. They claim the West is trying to pin the blame for AIDS on Africa, arguing that AIDS cannot be a serious problem in Nigeria when the only place where they see people with AIDS is in foreign documentaries on television.' (*WorldAIDS* Jan 1993:13)

Foreign media also bring Africa false messages which reinforce such denials of an epidemic. An extraordinary debate raged recently in the columns of the London *Sunday Times*' science correspondent, Neville Hodgkinson (e.g. 21 March 1993; 3 October 1993; 28 November 1993). It claimed that the African AIDS plague was a myth perpetuated by an AIDS establishment with a lot of money and political capital at stake. Some of the 'experts' interviewed argued that HIV positive tests were actually reactions to malaria 'producing up to 80–90% false positives.' (21 March 1993) (While early tests may have produced some false positives, today's tests, especially where a second method is used to confirm results, make such problems unlikely.) Others blamed increasing poverty, poor health care, the growth of drug-resistant strains of diseases such as malaria and tuberculosis and the growing use of drugs, such as smokeable heroin and cocaine, rather than HIV for the increasing morbidity and mortality in Africa. A handful of scientists claimed that HIV itself was harmless; it was merely a viral fellow-traveller in the bloodstreams of those already chronically ill or suffering multiple infections as a result of their lifestyles.

It is undoubtedly true that poverty and social disruption have aggravated health problems in Africa (see Chapter 4), and have generally been recognized as co-factors, hastening the onset of AIDS in those infected with HIV. Nevertheless those who work in Africa recognize that what is happening is not merely an increase of illness and death, but something of an entirely different order. Another major British newspaper, the *Independent on Sunday*, under the headline 'HIV is Africa's big killer', published rebuttals of the Hodgkinson articles by leading scientists, doctors and health organizations working in Africa. They claimed that Hodgkinson had distorted or disregarded scientific evidence, and that their letters to the paper were ignored or edited to reduce their impact or misrepresent their authors. *The Independent* quotes Spencer Haggard, chief executive of the Health Education Authority as saying the *Sunday Times*' approach "is akin to believing in medieval alchemy". (The *Independent on Sunday*, 14 November 1993) What could be the purpose of such "criminal misrepresentation?" Professor James Neil, a member of the British Medical Research Council's AIDS Steering Committee, accuses Hodgkinson of 'wilfully manufacturing controversy' to raise his own profile and that of his newspaper. (*The Argus* 15-12-1993) Given that people will jump at the chance to deny the existence of AIDS, and the need to modify their behaviour, large scale sowing of the seeds of denial on such fertile ground, by normally credible sources ranks as dangerously irresponsible.

The media debate is far from dead. The October 1994 issue of the African news magazine *New African*, managed to run two articles alongside each other, one citing a group of 'dissident scientists' who insist that AIDS is not caused by HIV, the other by 'eminent scientist', Dr Alan Cantwell Jr, who implies it was a man-made virus 'put into the human population as a genocidal agent for world population control' and 'a new and highly lethal microbiologic agent ... introduced into the black and gay populations in America.' (p.13) Such confusing contradictions, if taken seriously at a political level, militate against the chance of rational, concerted AIDS programmes in Africa.

The common perception that all of Africa is in the grip of an AIDS disaster has fuelled old racist patterns; they were reinforced by suggestions that Africans had 'caught' HIV from contact with the African green monkey, or, the more lurid version, that it came from bizarre sexual practices involving the monkey. At least 50 countries have insisted that immigrants, or foreign students or visitors coming for longer than a certain period be tested for HIV. In some cases, for instance Egypt, China, India, Belgium and Cyprus, these tests were apparently more stringently applied to Africans. (*WorldAIDS* March 1993:12; Waite 1988:155) Would-be blood donors from Africa or those who have visited Africa in the past seven years face rejection in America and Europe. African students in Moscow and Peking who used to hear 'monkey' called after them, might now hear '*spid*' and '*aizbig*', respectively the Russian and Chinese words for AIDS. (*New African* August 1990:41) Under the circumstances, it is hardly surprising that many African governments, certainly initially, were reluctant to admit to an epidemic. Rodger Yeager sums up the political significance of the issue: 'This reluctance to report AIDS cases results from African elites' unwillingness to have their countries viewed as cultural – and racial – pariahs of sexually communicated lethal disease. It also stems from a determination to protect foreign revenues, and from an equal fear of losing personal political legitimacy garnered through highly fragile patronage networks linking elites with each other and with their ethnic and sectional power bases.' (1988:73)

The blame and prejudice that have underpinned the growing racism, directed against Africa and immigrants in general, have also fuelled a growing homophobia. The initial link between AIDS and homosexuality led many Africans to deny that it would become an issue for them, since homosexuality was a 'Western problem'. Some African writers have even accused the Western gay community of trying to divert homophobia by backing the AIDS-and-Africa theories; Haitians in turn suggested that African monkeys imported as pets into homosexual brothels in Haiti had spread the virus. (Chirimuuta and Chirimuuta 1987:6) The desperate urge to foist the blame on others, shows the alarm homosexuals, Africans and immigrants have felt as they see this epidemic's stigmatizing potential undermining their fragile social status in many places.

Gay communities, at least in the industrialized countries, have been able to fight back against the disease and its social consequences with considerably more resources than most African and immigrant communities. The fact that AIDS was first diagnosed in the urban, educated, middle-class gay communities of the United States in the 1980s was crucial in the way the disease was perceived and treated. Another time, another place, another community would have produced very different responses. Indeed, it may have taken far longer for AIDS even to be identified as a new disease.

In the late 1970s for instance, injecting drug users had experienced a pneumonia outbreak which was probably HIV-related, but because they were seen as an intrinsically unhealthy community, the epidemic, labelled 'junkie pneumonia', passed largely unremarked. (Patton 1990:27–28) By contrast, the initial cluster of *Pneumocystis carinii* pneumonia among young male homosexuals in Los Angeles reported in 1981 set alarm bells ringing in the Centers for Disease Control (CDC) in Atlanta. Other rare conditions such as Kaposi's sarcoma, which caused purple skin lesions, and unusual lymph-cell cancers were also appearing in homosexual communities in American cities, and the CDC warned that a potential new epidemic was underway. Cindy Patton believes that it was because the men involved were perceived as 'previously healthy' that their condition was taken seriously.

'That gay men were seen as 'healthy' despite having a variety of treatable sexually transmitted diseases attested to the acceptance and positive valuation of gay men and their sexuality in the urban settings where these early cases were under study. Had these cases appeared fifty years ago, and had the homosexuality of the patients been recognized, doctors would probably have viewed homosexuals *per se* as constitutionally weaker and explained their immune system breakdown on this fact alone.' (Patton 1990:28) Pneumonia in drug users, or tuberculosis and diarrhoea in Africans would probably have needed to reach far more dramatic levels before a new causative factor was sought.

The timing of the AIDS epidemic also crucially affected the way the world has responded. Trends in the United States reflect this. Earlier US responses to epidemics such as cholera have not always been particularly sensitive to individual human rights. In the public uproar over the spread of venereal diseases early this century, for instance, 18,000 women suspected of prostitution were quarantined in state-run reformatories between 1918 and 1920. (Stoddard and Rieman 1991:241) Come the AIDS epidemic, there were the predictable calls for quarantine. So far the USA, and indeed most countries, with the highly-publicized exception of Cuba, have avoided quarantining the infected. Quarantine is only effective where diseases are easily identified, facilities are available and treatment can cure or ameliorate the condition. To test millions of healthy people and then incarcerate those infected for up to ten or fifteen years, is not socially or economically feasible. Despite the fact that research suggests up to 30% of Americans would like to see the HIV-infected quarantined, official responses have instead emphasized rational and compassionate programmes, voluntary cooperation rather than coercion, and the enactment of anti-discriminatory legislation. The most important reason for the changed approach probably lies in the law. As Thomas Stoddard and Walter Rieman point out, in the three decades between 1950 and 1980, civil rights and liberties 'received greater sustained attention than they had at any time since Reconstruction.' (1991:241–242) AIDS is the first health crisis of the post-civil rights revolution era, and with some exceptions (ibid.:263–266), responses to the epidemic have been influenced by this fact.

The civil rights movement coincided with the social revolutions of the 1960s and 1970s and a period of economic expansion. AIDS, by contrast, arrived at a time of economic recession and growing conservatism. Not only were they the years of Ronald Reagan and Margaret Thatcher, of 'family values' and the moral majority, but also a time in which the US Supreme Court was moving towards a majority of conservative justices. (ibid.:249) Despite this, as Stoddard and Rieman point out, 'while discrimination unquestionably exists, systematic attempts to deny employment, housing, goods or services to people with AIDS or HIV have been fewer than history would have led one to fear.' (ibid.:263)

Crucial to this tolerance – or at least lack of systematic discrimination – was the political strength of the gay movement particularly in the United States. Rooted in three decades of growing activism on behalf of homosexual rights, they faced what commentators immediately labelled 'the gay plague', with formidable strategic skill and commitment.

As the dimensions of the problem became clearer, and cases passed the thousand mark, gay activists in New York, Los Angeles and San Francisco debated the medical and political consequences of what they saw unfolding. In New York, an organization called Gay Men's Health Crisis was formed, to provide practical and political support for those affected. Other groups organized nationally. One of the first successes of these pressure groups was to persuade the CDC that the term they had coined for the syndrome, 'gay related immune deficiency', or GRID, was 'misleading and inappropriate' and the disease was renamed AIDS (Stoddard and Rieman 1991:256) – a term which not only proved to be more accurate, but surely spared the gay community at least some measure of homophobic responses.

Although the 1960s and 1970s had seen the decline of discrimination against homosexuals, many feared that the link between the AIDS epidemic and the gay community would rekindle the old prejudice; that the fear and abhorrence of AIDS would become fear and abhorrence of homosexuals. As Harvard's Allan Brandt explained: 'AIDS threatened the heterosexual culture with homosexual contamination. In this context, homosexuality – not a virus – causes AIDS. Therefore, homosexuality itself is feared as if it were a communicable, lethal disease. After a generation of work to have homosexuality removed as a disease from the psychiatric diagnostic manuals, it had suddenly reappeared as an infectious, terminal disease.' (1987:193)

The gay response to AIDS was multifold: defending the legal rights of infected people, lobbying to have the US Food and Drug Administration's rigorous drug-approval standards relaxed to allow the infected access to drugs which promised some hope in a hopeless landscape, monitoring medical and scientific developments, putting pressure on politicians and funders to increase the budgets for research and resources, raising public awareness of the threat, and, probably most significantly, developing *ad hoc*, but highly effective, campaigns to educate the gay community about safer sex, and to care for the hundreds, then thousands, then tens of thousands of gay men who became ill and ultimately helpless as the disease scythed its way through their communities. (For some accounts of the politics of AIDS in gay communities see e.g. Altman 1986, 1988; Carter and Watney (eds.) 1989; Daniel and Parker 1993; Kramer 1990; Patton 1990; Shilts 1987; Stoddard and Rieman 1991.)

The public response was in some ways paradoxical. AIDS increased the stigmatization of gays, but also forced public recognition of the movement and its demands. The adversarial stance between gay communities and the state which had characterized the 1960s and 1970s changed as the epidemic deepened. Gay demands for government-funded research, education and patient care meant that consultation and cooperation between their organizations and the state became necessary. Dennis Altman remarks on the irony that 'the conservative Reagan administration has had more contact with organized gay groups than any of its predecessors, largely because of AIDS.' (Altman 1988:302) It was not the only irony. New alliances with the state coincided with new enmities and divisions within the gay community itself. The bathhouses of San Francisco and New York, centres for the free-wheeling sexual encounters which had symbolized gay liberation, were closed amidst bitter debates about civil liberties, public health, and whether the AIDS scare was simply an enemy ploy to take away gay sexual freedom. (Shilts 1987)

Ultimately the programmes developed in the gay communities became models for state programmes, although gay social and cultural networks which facilitated the rapid diffusion of information and new safer sex practices, could not be reproduced in the heterogeneous communities of the wider United States, or elsewhere.

Dennis Altman talks of the effect of AIDS on the gay community as 'legitimation through disaster'. (1988) He argues that the response of governments in Western countries would have been 'very different – and almost certainly slower and more repressive' if the expanding gay networks of the 1970s 'had not also been accompanied by the growth of gay political organizations that provided a basis for the development of community-based groups in response to the epidemic .... AIDS has brought issues of central concern to the gay movement onto the mainstream political agenda: at an enormous price the gay movement has become a recognized actor in the politics of health policy-making.' (Altman 1988:313) It also demonstrated very clearly that the allocation of health resources is inherently political and responsive to effective lobbying.

The absorption of gay AIDS activists into the political mainstream has not universally been seen as a step forward. Writers such as Cindy Patton (1989, 1990) believe that the passion and commitment of the early activists and volunteer workers, who provided care and support for people with AIDS, were diverted into what Patton calls an 'AIDS service industry'. (Patton 1990:14) She believes that in the mid-1980s a major shift occurred '*away* from gay liberation-inspired resistance to a hostile government and indifferent medical empire, and *toward* an assimilation of activists into a new AIDS service industry, with its own set of commitments and its own structuring logic.' (ibid. – her emphasis)

The 'industry' was largely white and gay-community-based; increasingly it forsook its activist liberationist roots for bureaucratized, well-funded respectability (ibid. 1990:19–20; see also Kobasa 1991). In the process, its relevance to other people afflicted by the epidemic dwindled. Patton accuses the 'industry' of racism, classism and sexism, which has effectively prevented 'natural allies from forming coalitions in order to address problems raised by the HIV epidemic.' (1990:6)

Gay activists could become victims of their own political success. With their high political profile and their skills in applying pressure, gay needs have tended to overshadow those of the communities where

68

HIV is now spreading fastest in the United States – among injecting drug users and the poor, particularly blacks and Latinos. These communities do not have the same resources, either to fend for themselves or to apply pressure on the authorities for assistance.

Projects like Shanti, San Francisco's largest, and primarily gay-based, AIDS service organization, have been accused of discriminating against non-gay sufferers. In April 1988, the San Francisco Human Rights Commission actually filed a formal complaint against the Shanti project for possible discrimination against women and ethnic minorities. (Grover 1989:149) There is also a danger that if the AIDS lobby itself is sufficiently strong and manages to prioritize the needs of PWAs for housing and medical care or the care of AIDS orphans, this might increase resentment and prejudice against them, particularly in countries where need is ubiquitous. Special pleading by any group could open it to increased discrimination, and undermine attempts to build solidarity among all the afflicted. (See e.g. *AIDS in the World* pp. 675, 773, 795, 798)

That gays were in the vanguard of the AIDS counter-offensive is not in dispute. However, as the epidemic spreads, there is growing criticism that they are exploiting the AIDS issue to advance the gay cause and recruit homosexuals who might previously not have aligned themselves with the movement. Others are concerned that even if the gay epidemic declines, this powerful constituency could ensure that funds would continue to be channelled to gay-specific programmes at the expense of other vulnerable people.

In their turn, gay activists such as Dennis Altman have complained that the epidemic has been 'de-gayed' by those governments or organizations which were either unwilling to be seen supporting a predominantly gay cause, or by AIDS organizations which were under

'considerable political pressure ... to de-emphasize their gay identity.'
(*AIDS in the World* 1992:388–9) Recent research in many countries
suggests that after the early successful response of the gay communities to their own safer sex campaigns, there is a dangerous and growing trend to ignore the message, particularly among gay adolescents,
who did not witness the carnage of the first wave of the epidemic; 'de-
gaying' the epidemic might make it particularly hard to educate a new
generation who see AIDS as a disease of 'old gays'.

Recently, too, gay leadership has been accused of neglecting AIDS
issues in favour of pushing a broader political agenda, taking up issues
such as the rights of gay couples or gays in the military. Outspoken
activist Larry Kramer reflects that gay organizations are involved in
bruising fights for funds and constituents. Apart from such 'territorial
infighting' gay organizations all 'seem eventually to fall victim to
endemic bitchiness and bitterness.' (1990:252)

Kramer, himself a co-founder of the GMHC, deplored the bureaucrat-
ization, the 'taming' of the organization over the years and, in 1987,
founded ACT-UP (the AIDS Coalition to Unleash Power), a band of
political activists 'too angry simply to sit down with [President]
George Bush.' (Kobasa 1991:182) Not a service organization, ACT-
UP uses challenge and confrontation as its strategies – public demon-
strations, street theatre, civil disobedience, 'happenings' – to focus
public and government attention on the AIDS crisis.

There has also been criticism of the gay community's heavy emphasis
on less stringent testing and free availability of new, potentially useful
drugs. While a man with five years to live cannot wait eight years for
the Food and Drug Administration to approve a drug, is he justified in
demanding its immediate release? Robert Gallo writes:

I cannot think of a more sharply two-edged sword: the faster drugs are moved into therapy the greater the risk of incompetence, serious toxic side effects, even outright fraud. Numerous treatments for AIDS have raised instant headlines, caused harm, then disappeared. Those who sped them into clinical use by vocal support of 'activism', then simply stopped talking about them. (1991:234)

Gallo also points out that not all activists fall into this category; he singles out Martin Delaney's Project Inform as an intelligent, well-informed organization providing accurate information to thousands of HIV-infected people with its publications. Whatever the criticisms of gay AIDS activism in the United States may be, they have certainly demonstrated that a well-organized, highly motivated and articulate lobby can actually change the balance of power between patients and the medical establishment.

Gay communities outside the United States have had varied success in dealing with AIDS through self-empowerment and political leverage. In Australia, where by 1993, 87% of AIDS cases still resulted from male-to-male transmission, the majority of infections occurred in identifiable gay communities, according to Gary Dowsett of the National Centre for HIV Social Research at Macquarie University, Sydney. After 1984 when the epidemic began to grow rapidly, a comprehensive programme was instituted, involving cooperation and consultation between all levels of government, public health officials, non-governmental organizations (initially and predominantly gay communities), health professionals and academics. From the outset this involved major government funding of gay community agencies and programmes. Dowsett believes the decreasing rate of new HIV infection over more than five years can be attributed to a strong, established gay community with international links and information resources, and to

71

its willingness to develop and respond to the AIDS programmes. Important, too, was their recognition that there were men engaged in sex with men, on an occasional or commercial basis, but not part of the gay scene, who needed education from the gay organizations. (WHO/ GPA 1993:25)

British gay organizations have compared their lot unfavourably with those of their USA counterparts. AIDS activist Simon Watney concedes that 'the government's AIDS education programme has reflected a low-profile anti-interventionist neo-liberal school of thought, rather than the aggressive moralism of its neo-conservative wing.' (Watney 1989:21) Nevertheless, there has been censorship of education materials which did not adopt a moral position or support 'family values', or promoted homosexual relationships as acceptable.

At the 1987 Conservative Party conference, Prime Minister Margaret Thatcher had protested: "Children who need to be taught to respect traditional moral values are being taught that they have an inalienable right to be gay." (Watney 1989:23) Watney accuses the British government of 'not spending a single penny on directly communicating support, sympathy or information' (ibid.:25) to the gay community. That government AIDS spending was less than lavish, was in part a consequence of the belt-tightening in the British health budget of the day. While critics would agree with Watney on the insufficiency of funding, many nevertheless approved of the low-key, anti-discriminatory tone of the British response and its avoidance of the hysteria which marked some elements in the United States' responses. (Porter and Porter 1988:114-115) The British government recognized the very valuable role of the voluntary sector. In January 1988, in a report by the Social Services Committee of the Department of Health and Social Security, it acknowledged that educational material, particularly where it was very explicit, was often best put across by bodies already active in specific communities such as gay or ethnic groups. (1988:10) The government also recognized that 'AIDS raises complex moral, social and ethical questions,' and while celibacy before marriage and fidelity within it were the best way of avoiding HIV, it recognized that 'this advice may not be acceptable to all groups and particularly some of those most at risk.' (1988:11) The safer sex message, including public advertizing of condoms was therefore accepted. (ibid.)

Western European states, which began reporting AIDS cases shortly after the United States, estimated cumulative HIV infections of 720,000 in 1992, compared with the 1,180,000 in the United States. (*AIDS in the World* 1992:27) France, with an incidence of 403 per million population, and Switzerland, with 413 per million, were the worst affected. Campaigns have recognized that non-discrimination is a central issue in any successful programme. In October 1989, the Council of Europe declared that there should be explicit policy commitments to the rights of HIV-infected individuals 'to enjoy the same civil and social rights as the non-infected, while bearing ethical, civil and legal responsibilities to contain transmission.' (*AIDS in the World* 1992:561) Nevertheless reports of discriminatory practices by, for instance, insurance companies, employers, medical practitioners and educational institutions are common. Gay communities, which have everywhere in Europe been among the worst affected by the epidemic, have campaigned against discrimination. Given their organization and the strengths of their support networks, they are often in a better position to protest than, for instance, drug users or prostitutes who lack the political skills or who fear still further stigmatization if they speak out.

Public policies in Europe may outlaw actual discrimination, but prejudice persists. Research suggests that while most people would stop short of joining right-wing thugs in attacks on gays or their property, attitudes are far from universally tolerant. In West Germany, for instance, the trend towards increasing tolerance of homosexuality, apparent in the 1970s, reversed in the 1980s. Younger respondents, particularly, were likely to make moral judgements on homosexuality, and AIDS appeared to underlie this change. (Hessling and Heckman 1993:64) In one study of 2118 adults, 59.6% agreed that so-called 'high-risk groups' (of which gays would be a significant part) have to be blamed for the spread of AIDS. (ibid.:112) In a study of 2387 Danish students aged 13 to 20, 37% thought HIV-positive people should be registered, 56% that they should live in celibacy and 24% that they should be isolated. (ibid.:145)

Elsewhere in the world, homosexuals have had very mixed fortunes as the epidemic tightens its grip on their communities. The organized and militant gay communities of America and Europe often do not exist in developing countries. In places such as Pakistan, where homosexuality is 'rampant' (*WorldAIDS* January 1993:11) there is no gay community in the Western sense of the word. In a society where men and women are segregated by custom, men may use other men to satisfy their sexual needs, despite the laws that forbid this. A majority of these men do not regard themselves as homosexual. It is a puritanical society; there is no attempt at state education. Informed gays, who try to educate those they believe are at risk, are ignored. As one gay doctor remarked: "You cannot teach safe sex in a society which refuses to acknowledge its own sexuality." (ibid.)

It is important, too, to realize that homosexuals are nowhere a homogeneous group. To some extent, the idea of 'the gay community' has been a political construct of the gay liberation movement, which gave structure and power to their organizations. As in Pakistan, many men who have sex with men do not see themselves as homosexual, much less part of a 'gay' sub-culture. In Mexico, such men may regard gay men much as heterosexuals often do – as degenerate or abnormal.

74

Stigmatized Victims: risk, blame and discrimination

Juan Hernandez, a Mexican gay activist, noted further complexities, such as gay men rejecting bisexuals, and divisions between 'effeminate young men, transvestites and older, macho gay men.' *(WorldAIDS* March 1993:2) In Mexico such discord makes it difficult to devise appropriate education strategies, and he sees little progress in gay human rights:

> ... overall, the prevailing response is sex-negative, prejudiced and – perhaps most worryingly – violent. Even though increasingly larger segments of society are willing to view homosexuals in a more positive light, abuse, discrimination, assaults and even murders are normal responses to the popular association between AIDS and homosexuality. (ibid.)

Most research data on AIDS and homosexuality is fragmentary. An exception is the book by Herbert Daniel and Richard Parker *Sexuality, Politics and AIDS in Brazil* (1993) which explores the epidemic in its social, political and cultural context. I have said, in talking of the epidemics in South Africa and the United States, that their time and place of arrival was crucial to the nature of the responses they generated. Daniel and Parker make the same points for Brazil. The late 1980s was a period of growing political and economic pessimism which eroded the earlier hopes of a return to a civilian society, in which individual citizens and non-government organizations could influence the political process. The nascent gay movement was stifled, and as AIDS took hold, homosexuals experienced growing discrimination and even violence against them, including police persecution in the name of AIDS prevention. (ibid.:23) The government, facing enormous health and social problems, financially weak, and hesitant to offend the Roman Catholic Church, did little to inform the public. By 1994 the Catholic Church in Brazil, as elsewhere, continued to ban the use of condoms.

75

HAROLD BRIDGES LIBRARY
S. MARTIN'S COLLEGE
LANCASTER

Homosexual and bisexual Brazilians were hard-hit by the epidemic, but lacked the strong gay community organization of Western countries. Daniel talks of the difficulties of AIDS education in Brazil, '[w]here even today it has to be proven, even to gay men, that there is such a thing as an AIDS epidemic, and not just a CIA plot to wipe out all gays, or a device of the newspapers to encourage their persecution.' (Daniel and Parker 1993:46)

In the face of government inaction and a growing Brazilian epidemic – from 32 AIDS cases in 1983 to more than 26,000 in 1991 – new organizations, to educate the public and to care for and defend the rights of those infected, began to emerge. Daniel and Parker speak of 'a politics of AIDS aimed at confronting not only the epidemics of HIV infection and AIDS, but also the third epidemic of prejudice and blame.' (1993:60) In a society where authoritarian rule had progressively weakened the institutions of civil society, Daniel and Parker find it heartening that associations of gays, of church people, of medical practitioners and intellectuals should be coming together to deal with the scourge, to destroy it as 'a disease of hopelessness.' (1993:134)

The AIDS pandemic, by virtue of the major targets it has picked – homosexuals, drug addicts, prostitutes, immigrants, the poor, 'foreigners' – has immensely complicated the world's responses. There is a haunting question at the heart of the pandemic: if AIDS had struck first at millions of young, white, straight, middle-class American or European men, would we be any closer to a solution? Probably not, but that does not stop those who have suffered, first the stigmatization and marginalization of the contemporary world, and now this fiendish disease, from asking the question.

CHAPTER 4

THE SAVAGERY OF LIFE: POWERLESSNESS AND VULNERABILITY

The critical factors in controlling the epidemic do not lie among people who can make choices, but rather among those who cannot – especially the poorest, least powerful, most vulnerable and most isolated.
(Klouda 1992:797)

In *Ground Zero*, author Andrew Holleran equates the effects of the AIDS epidemic on American gays with the terror of the French Revolution; for the first time they came face to face with the 'savagery of life' which middle class Americans had always been spared. (1988:14) Not all AIDS' targets have been that lucky. Increasingly, those affected are the poor in urban ghettos, illegal migrants, drug users, street children, prostitutes, or the impoverished people in Third World countries. They are not unacquainted with the savagery of life. For them, AIDS is just an additional problem, often faced with their customary fatalism. Fatalism is no protection against AIDS. To protect

themselves against this new threat, they must know the facts and practise safer sex; but, as Klouda says, the poor, the powerless, the isolated, the vulnerable, do not control these choices. Their access to facts
and their ability to practise safer sex are compromised by the circumstances of their lives.

They do not control the political process, the policy-making or the
resources which, as the earlier chapters explain, provide the founda-
tions for self-protection and care. They are easy prey for AIDS, which
travels along societies' faultlines, exploiting weakness and instability.
The history of the HI virus is still far from clear. What is clear is that
wherever it may have lurked before, the last three decades have created ideal environments for it to surface in epidemic form. They have
been decades of rapid social change, of urbanization and changing
norms and values, of population explosions, of environmental and
political disasters, of increasing poverty and disadvantage and social
disintegration. Guenter Risse writes that to understand why diseases
appear, how they spread and why they depart, you have to understand
the 'dynamic relationship between the biosocial environment and
humans – an "ecology' of disease". (Risse 1988:33) Although the circumstances in the homosexual and heterosexual epidemics appear different, in fact they are 'ecologically' similar.

Since the 1960s both the Western gay communities and increasingly
people in the developing world, have slipped their old cultural moor-
ings and been swept along in the rapid currents of contemporary
change. Andrew Holleran, writing of the American gay sub-culture in
the 1970s, equates the freewheeling sex of the time with liberation:
'Rubbers were jokes, the idea of constraints on sex anathema to those
who argued that the essence of sex was freedom, and the glory of freedom sex ... safety ran counter to the whole expansive spirit of the sev-
enties, the exhilarating suspicion that we were pioneers in the pursuit

of human happiness and no one had found its limits yet. The plague provided limits.' (1988:24)

Holleran makes Risse's connection – that sexual freedom helps create the habitat for plague. The same breakdown of constraints is at work elsewhere in the world. In the developing world, it is tied not only to rapid urbanization, but to the 'modernization' of norms and values which accompanies the accelerating process. Post-colonial Africa has been particularly affected. In his examination of poverty in Africa, Anthony O'Connor notes that 'along with general population growth, one of the greatest changes taking place across tropical Africa from the 1960s to the 1980s has been the world's highest *rate* of urbanization.' (1991:44 – his emphasis)

How do these developments create a disease 'ecology', a situation where the virus can flourish? AIDS in the developing world is predominantly a sexually transmitted disease. Apart from north-east Asia and the south-east Mediterranean, where injecting drug use is also significant and accounts for about 20% of infections, the vast majority of transmissions are sexual. In Latin America, homosexual relations still accounted for the majority of infections (54%) in a 1992 survey, but heterosexual transmission predominated in sub-Saharan Africa (93%), the Caribbean (75%), Southeast Asia (70%) and north-east Asia (50%). (*AIDS in the World* 1992:32)

The effective sexual transmission of HIV – or indeed any STD – depends on the level of infection – or seroprevalence – in the community, and the level of unprotected sexual activity. The density of sexual networks increases with, for instance, the density of population, the percentage of that population which is in the most sexually active cohort (say, 15 to 35 years old), the male to female ratio, the absence, or marginalization, of those who would normally enforce conservative sexual values, and the positive evaluation of the 'pursuit of human happiness'. The characteristics of the world's gay capitals and many of the rapidly urbanizing centres of the developing world, encouraged high levels of sexual activity – not for everyone in them, of course, but enough to create a *Zeitgeist* very congenial to the flourishing of HIV.

None of this should be read as moral criticism; the changing mores were a predictable result of the social dynamics and the demographic trends of the time. In the burgeoning towns and cities of the developing world, population growth has been driven both by internal growth (itself partly a result of the relatively youthful nature of its populace) and accelerating in-migration from rural areas. Urban populations have growth at twice the rate of those in the countryside. (Tolley and Thomas 1987:1) Migration has been fuelled by both urban 'pull' and rural 'push' factors. The lure of towns – as places to make a new start, to accumulate wealth, to escape the mundane village world – has probably been less significant for the majority of migrants than the need to escape the poverty of overcrowded and deteriorating farms, to earn cash to send home to keep the rural family viable, or to finance health, education or bridewealth needs.

When people migrate to town they seldom cut their rural ties entirely. Some alternate periods as migrant labourers with time back in the countryside. For others, there is inevitably a coming and going between places – going home to visit family, to find a country wife, to take part in important rituals, to consult family elders or traditional healers, or to have a baby, to spend holidays, convalesce, retire or die. Together with links of trade, administration and services, this rural–urban shuttle carries HIV from the cities into even the most remote locations.

In the short run, the most dangerous migrations, in terms of disease ecology, are those precipitated by natural and man-made disasters. Great tracts of the Third World, in Latin America, Asia, the Middle East and particularly Africa, are crisscrossed with the paths of people fleeing drought and famine, civil war and political disorder. In 1991, the US Committee for Refugees estimated that 15 million people were refugees in foreign lands, and another 15 to 20 million were internal refugees in their own countries. (Brogan 1992:viii) Whether they seek sanctuary in town, village, neighbouring country or refugee camp they are uniquely vulnerable, cut loose from the structures and values that supported and constrained them. Add to that a sense of hopelessness or fatalism, and 'safe sex' may be the last thing on the refugee's mind. As Dr Santiago Almeida, chief epidemiologist in El Salvador's Public Health Ministry noted: "People in El Salvador are used to death. When you lose over 70,000 people to a 10-year civil war ... it's tough to convince people that AIDS prevention should be their utmost concern." (*WorldAIDS* July 1991:3) During the war, nearly one-fifth of El Salvador's population migrated to the United States, fleeing the war and the economic crisis. Many have since returned infected with HIV, or were infected by the growing prostitution that accompanied the war. (ibid.) That soldiers and prostitutes are fellow-travellers is as old as military history. So is the coincidence of war with disease, in populations raped, uprooted and left destitute in its wake.

Africa has been particularly ill-fated insofar as the onset of AIDS and a period of widespread instability have coincided. In the years since AIDS came to Africa, war and political violence in Angola, Burundi, Rwanda, Ethiopia, Liberia, Mozambique, Namibia, Somalia, South Africa, Sudan and Uganda have cost millions of lives and forced countless millions to flee.

Wars and anarchy create ideal conditions for the transmission of HIV. Soldiers and civilians, many moving without partners or families for extended periods, live outside of conventional morality; many resort to prostitution to satisfy their needs. In Ethiopia, for instance, years of civil war, compounded by drought and famine, have spread HIV throughout the country. AIDS experts estimate that up to 15% of the sexually active population are infected. Another legacy of the war is the estimated 500,000 prostitutes; in Addis Ababa, research suggests that 95% of the prostitutes are HIV positive (*WorldAIDS* Sept 1993:11)

In 1992, the city of Juba in Southern Sudan, which had a population of 36,000 people 9 years previously at the start of the civil war, grew to 500,000. Sex was a taboo topic for discussion, but it thrived in the crowded city. 'Most of the women diagnosed with HIV or AIDS in Juba are age 14–20, separated from their families by the war and driven into prostitution in order to survive.' (*WorldAIDS* Sept 1992:10)

War brutalizes human relationships. Rape and the sexual abuse of women, children and even men flourishes; in Bosnia, Rwanda, Mozambique, everywhere, in fact, war brings sexual violence in its wake. 'For many civilian women, it is hard to refuse sex to a soldier wielding a gun.' (*WorldAIDS* Nov1992:5)

War spreads AIDS in other ways – emergency blood transfusions in the field may use any volunteer blood offered, without testing. Because of their accessibility, soldiers are often called on as donors despite the fact that they commonly register very high infection rates. In Lebanon, doctors worry that blood imported during the years of civil war has been responsible for infections. Health services suffer; STDs, which facilitate HIV transmission, are left untreated, AIDS programmes collapse, and preventive care, necessary to stem the tide of infectious diseases that endanger HIV positive people, breaks down. The physical and psychological battering of war, stresses people's immune systems further. Countries that offer sanctuary may also be at risk. In Malawi, itself one of the worst affected countries, nearly 10% of the population are Mozambican refugees, who have fled the civil war since it began in 1976. There is great concern that 'this million-strong exiled community, suffering physical and psychological after-shocks of war, face additional barriers to responsible sexual behaviour and change.' (*WorldAIDS* March 1992:9) After the 1994 Rwandan massacres, hundreds of thousands of Rwandans fled into neighbouring Zaire and Tanzania. Desperate relief agencies battled to prevent the outbreak of cholera and typhoid in the refugee camps; in the crisis of the moment, little thought could be given to AIDS prevention in what *WorldAIDS* has referred to as 'one of Africa's hottest AIDS spots.' (Sept 1994:1) In the Zairean camps, flooded with over two million refugees, cholera broke out and tens of thousands died. To use scarce resources on AIDS education in such circumstances might strike the refugees as little short of grotesque.

The legacies of these wars will be felt in growing numbers of AIDS cases for years to come, and sometimes in social changes that will last still longer. 'Sex tourism' is a case in point. The current thriving industry in Southeast Asia 'derived much of its momentum from the war in Vietnam, where impoverished young women from the coun-tryside flocked to military centers to service visiting troops on "rest and relaxation".' (*AIDS in the World* 1992:182) It is perhaps in war that politics most clearly appears as the handmaiden of AIDS.

War and the flight of refugees offer extreme versions of the conditions facing ordinary migrants. They, too, are cut loose from the supports and constraints of their home communities. Whether rural sexual norms were impossibly prim and rigid, or relaxed and free-and-easy, the town will inevitably confront the new migrant with choices. Freed from the surveillance and sanctions of the village he or she will be faced with a *smörgäsbord* of behavioural options. Some migrants may opt to recreate rural patterns, deliberately building networks of people who share these values, but many will browse through the mix-and-match options on offer – anything from anonymous sexual encounters, to a whole variety of commercial sex transactions from the one-night stand, to domestic service, including sexual favours, to varieties of concubinage, to formal marriage.

The penalties and rewards that reinforced village patterns change or fall away. For instance, the unmarried girl who became pregnant would have been ostracized by her peers in the village; the man responsible would have been expected to pay a fine. In the city their behaviour may hardly cause a raised eyebrow. The man who fails to support the child he fathered, may not only go unpunished, but actually find his macho image enhanced. There has been much debate about 'promiscuity' as the root cause of HIV spread, particularly in Africa; it must always be seen against this background of rapid urbanization and the erosion of traditional social systems. Such systems, while they may not have measured up to missionary requirements, ensured that sexual behaviour was everywhere subject to a set of rules designed to protect the social fabric. Viewed in normative and structural terms, today's cities are not so much social fabric as patchwork quilt. Creating coherent and credible AIDS programmes in such hetero-geneous and fluid communities is highly problematic.

A major dimension of the AIDS risk in rapidly growing cities is pover-ty. The poverty which drives people out of the rural areas may be greater in absolute terms than that of the urban areas, but for the migrant, the struggle may seem no easier than the one he or she left behind; the load of the second or third generation urbanite may be only marginally better. The new, raw cities of the world are an assault, not only on the migrants' beliefs and values, but also on their physical well-being. Unless they are part of a very fortunate minority, perhaps with urban relatives already established, they will scrabble to find even rudimentary accommodation, as the shacklands surrounding Third World cities attest. Although a shack may represent the first step on the ladder to becoming urban, it is a dangerous and rickety foothold, not least in health terms. This is not unique to the Third World. A glance at life in nineteenth century London reveals a growing, industrializing city that would be recognizable in today's developing world.

> On entering these houses you have a fine specimen of the manner in which the lower orders of Westminster live. Living by day and night in one wretched room, with scarcely any light – an intermittent supply of water, and a shocking faetid atmosphere – full of rags and filth – it is dreadful! In the corner of the room may be seen what may be termed an apology for a bed and bedding, being a mass of rags piled together, in the midst of which are the poor sickly children, whose very countenance bespeak that they will soon cease to trouble their parents; with hair uncombed, barefooted and in rags – with their skin unwashed – the majority of them never live to manhood, while one third of them die before they attain the age of 5 years. The adult inhabitants, also, have all the appearance of being always in a typhoid state. The courts and alleys in this colony of filth and fever are chiefly unpaved and undrained, and mostly with but one privy for one court, which contains, sometimes upward of twenty houses. (Quoted in Sanders and Carver 1985:25)

I quote this description at some length not just because the picture is so strikingly familiar, or because it is salutary to remember how recently much of the First World lived in Third World conditions, but also because the authors' prescription for change is germane to the argument of this chapter – that for health to improve, politics must change. Sanders and Carver note that poor nutrition and a plethora of infectious diseases made the onslaughts on nineteenth-century health in Europe very much like those in today's developing countries. The majority of Europeans died of airborne diseases such as TB, pneumonia, diphtheria, measles and scarlet fever, or water-and food-related diseases such as diarrhoea, dysentery and cholera. Non-respiratory TB, often contracted from drinking infected milk, or insect-borne diseases, such as typhus and plague, were also essentially products of living conditions.

They describe the rapid improvement in health in the hundred years from 1870 to 1970. In 1870, infant mortality was 160 per 1000 live births; by 1900 it had dropped to 140, by 1920 to 80, by 1950 to 30 and by 1970 to less than 20. (ibid.:28) 'Modern medicine' is commonly credited with these advances, but the authors point out that, in fact, the most important forces behind the changes were improved living conditions and better hygiene, particularly clean water, sanitation, and better nutrition – essentially products of improved public health policy and practices. Specific preventive measures, such as smallpox vaccine, and, much later, anti-bacterial drugs, played a secondary role. (ibid.:36)

HIV differs from the great killers of nineteenth-century Europe, insofar as it is sexually, rather than environmentally, transmitted. Poor health and living conditions, and particularly untreated STDs, nevertheless make people more vulnerable to HIV infection, and accelerate the progression to full-blown AIDS. Such an environment also provides a rich brew of potential opportunistic infections to afflict people with depleted immune systems. Given that modern medicine has not yet produced the 'magic bullet' that will cure or prevent AIDS, public health policy and education are critical. The poor, the powerless and the vulnerable will need particular attention – not only carefully targeted education programmes, but also attention to mopping up all the curable and preventable conditions such as TB, STDs, hepatitis B, and poor nutrition which flourish in poverty, and precipitate AIDS deaths.

It is a debatable issue whether such policies will be forthcoming. Health budgets are very much at the mercy of politics. In her analysis of women's health in Africa, political scientist Meredeth Turshen comments: 'Medical technology develops with a logic of its own, independent of the population's needs; it serves the government and its influential medical corps as an instrument of power.' (Turshen 1991:207) She points to the expensive research centre built in Gabon to study fertility problems as an example. 'While sexually transmitted diseases go untreated and the infant mortality rate hovers above one hundred per thousand live births, the government is reinforcing its popularity by catering to urban elites concerned with low birth rates.' (ibid.)

For governments wishing to enhance their public image, the media event surrounding a successful heart transplant, a life saved, is worth far more than the invisible tally of deaths prevented by humble primary health care. As Reginald Green points out, politicians around the world 'relate to what they perceive to be the needs and demands of those to whom they are accountable or toward whom they feel responsible.... Most politicians in the South are not very effectively accountable to poor people (by elections or otherwise) and many do not feel responsible to or for them. Few actually practise trying to find out how poor people perceive their own needs, or how they would prefer to be empowered to meet them.' (1991:751)

There is a school of thought that defines AIDS unequivocally as 'a disease of poverty', a modern equivalent of nineteenth-century TB, and that believes the solution will come with a fairer economic dispensation. As the discussion so far suggests, poverty undoubtedly aids and abets HIV. But ultimately it produces epidemics only in conjunction with the virus itself, and a complex alignment of behavioural, cultural, social, political and economic conditions. Poverty alone is not a sufficient condition. The Western epidemics did not start among the under-privileged, although they have since battened on the poor and marginalized. In Africa, too, the early victims were not the poorest or most vulnerable. (Miller and Rockwell 1988:Introduction) In Malawi, for instance, a research team investigating risk factors for HIV infection among 5500 pregnant women, of whom 23% proved to be infected, found the main predictor for HIV seemed to be the higher socio-economic status of the husband or partner. (*WorldAIDS* March 1992:9) While some of the evidence from Africa is contradictory, it seems that, at least initially, infection was highest in 'the more wealthy and privileged groups,' whose relative affluence allowed them mobility, more disposable income, and greater access to 'beer and sex, with obvious implications for the spread of HIV.' (Whiteside 1993:228) More affluent communities are, however, also more likely to react to AIDS messages and modify their behaviour, or to have the resources to maximize available medical care and ensure that they enjoy the longest asymptomatic period after infection. The developing pandemic will increasingly confirm Renée Sabatier's description of AIDS as a 'misery-seeking missile.' (1988)

Nowhere is this analysis more potently demonstrated than with the two categories of people universally the poorest and most vulnerable of the poor and vulnerable – the women and children of Third World countries.

In First World countries, the panic about heterosexual transmission and the spread of AIDS into 'the wider community' has died down in the last few years. Partly this stems from better AIDS education and the reassuring message that people can protect themselves, but perhaps more significant are the statistical data. In Europe, heterosexual transmission dropped from 18% of all infections in 1985 to 10% in 1990; for women the drop was 54% to 30%. (Homosexual and bisexual transmission also dropped – from 63% in 1985 to 47% in 1990, but there has been alarming growth among injecting drug users. 30% of 1990 transmissions were by this method, as against only 5% in 1985.) Although heterosexual transmission has grown more rapidly in the USA – from 3% in 1985 to 7% in 1990 (*AIDS in the World* 1992:120) to 9% in 1993 (*MMWR* 3(9) March 1994 154–157), even there the nightmare scenarios of a wildfire spread have not been realized.

Significantly much of the increase in First World countries has been in their own 'Third World' sectors – their poorest, least powerful, most marginalized communities. In the United States two out of three adults living below the poverty level in 1983 were women (Panos 1990b:73) and the majority of women with HIV/AIDS are now black or Hispanic. (ibid.:41) The danger in this trend is that those with the power to make policies and allocate resources might designate AIDS one of 'their' diseases, not affecting 'us', and choose to ignore it, or greatly down-grade AIDS budgets. The more conservative the government, the more likely this is to happen.

The trend towards the 'feminization' of poverty is universal, but most acutely felt among the women, particularly rural women, in the poorest Third World countries. It is here that AIDS has cut deepest. By 1992, of the 11.8 million adults believed to be HIV-infected, 40% or 4.7 million, were women. Nearly 4 million of these women lived in sub-Saharan Africa. (*AIDS in the World* 1992:30) The growing epidemic among women in turn produces a paediatric epidemic as women pass the virus to their unborn or breast-feeding babies.

Why are women particularly at risk in the epidemic? And why is the vulnerability of poor women greater still?

women

Biology and socio-cultural forces both conspire against them. In the act of sexual intercourse women are exposed to greater concentrations of semen than men are to vaginal fluids. This fact alone multiplies women's risks, perhaps as much as tenfold, (Crewe 1993:28) Where women engage in anal intercourse whether for erotic or contraceptive reasons, the danger of infection is still greater. In African countries, where 83% of the world's infected women live, women also tend to become infected younger than men because men choose partners younger than themselves. AIDS, and the search for 'safe' partners, has skewed this pattern further. Alan Fleming notes: 'Transmission of HIV to females in Africa is largely a phenomenon of adolescence, but AIDS is a disease of young adulthood, with a peak of frequency coinciding with the age when women are most often pregnant.' (1993:297)

Avoiding pregnancy brings its own risks. The contraceptive pill and injection can both cause cervical inflammation and bleeding. Intra-uterine devices (IUDs) increase pelvic inflammatory diseases and possible localized cervical irritation. (Panos 1990b:16) In lives where poor health is normal, women often tolerate such discomforts, as they do a whole range of STDs, which often go untreated, even unnoticed. All of these conditions could facilitate HIV transmission.

Certain sexual practices, such as the preference for 'dry sex', or female circumcision, may also increase risks. To achieve dry sex, women use a variety of agents which are designed to tighten the vagina and dry up its natural secretions – everything from herbs to aluminium hydroxide, rock salt, stones or cloth. Information is still incomplete, but there is some evidence of such practices from widely separated areas – Malawi, Cameroon, Ghana, Kenya, Saudi Arabia, Haiti, Costa Rica, the Dominican Republic, Zaire, Zambia and Zimbabwe. Both mechanical and chemical methods could cause inflammation, lesions and the danger of haemorrhages, with consequent susceptibility to HIV and other infections. If dry sex is the cultural preference, the use of condoms which require lubrication would also be unpopular. (*WorldAIDS* May 1994:5–6) Female 'circumcision' is a term which covers practices ranging from a small symbolic nick on the thigh or clitoris, to genital mutilation in which substantial parts of the external female genitalia are removed, and the vulva stitched partly closed. It has the potential to facilitate HIV transmission both during the operation and through consequent complications during intercourse and childbirth. Fortunately, alarms about such practices raised early on in the epidemic have not been realized. The very young age of the girls involved (usually 5 to 8 years) makes cross-infection unlikely, and the areas where the most radical forms are practised, such as northern Sudan, southern Egypt and Somalia, are sexually conservative countries, as evinced by low rates of STDs, and HIV is, as yet, spreading slowly. (Taverne 1994:5–6; *WorldAIDS* May 1994:5–9) Male circumcision, which is known to give some protection against other STDs, may do the same with HIV, but operations carried out on a number of boys or young men at the same ceremony with non-sterile instruments, could equally spread infection if any of the initiates is HIV positive.

Hard data on whether pregnancy, which anyway taxes women's immune systems, precipitates AIDS in those who are HIV positive, are still not available. Some evidence suggests it may do so as a co-factor where the woman is also a drug addict, or suffers from malnutrition, other infections or parasites. (Panos 1990b:42; *AIDS in the World* 1992:640–641) Pregnancy and childbirth undoubtedly do expose women to additional HIV risks, particularly in developing countries where ante-natal health care is poor. Mothers often produce their first child at a very young age. Evert Ketting writes: 'More than 50 per cent of women in sub-Saharan Africa and Latin America give birth before the age of 20, ... [and] pregnancy-related complications are the major cause of death among girls in their late teens.' (1993:28) Anaemia, and blood loss during childbirth, which require transfusions in situations where HIV sero-prevalence is high and blood safety uncertain, pose immediate threats, but the medical procedures preceding, during and after childbirth, and throughout women's whole reproductive careers, especially where unsterile instruments or syringes are used, put them at far greater risk of medical transmission than most men experience.

What is certain, too, is that mothers can pass the virus on to their unborn babies either *in utero*, during birth or during breast-feeding. It is difficult to determine at birth whether the child has been affected since all babies will carry the antibodies passed on by the mother. Their own antibody reaction can only generally be tested with any level of accuracy from about 15 to 18 months of age, although newer, more sensitive – and often more costly and time-consuming – methods are available in sophisticated medical laboratories. (*AIDS in the World* 1992:632–634)

What are the risks of mother–child transmission? The information available at present suggests that the answer may again be a factor of the mother's circumstances. Studies from the United States, Canada, Haiti, Europe and a number of African countries have produced results as low as 7% (Spain) and as high as 42% (Congo). (The results need to be interpreted with caution as the survey subjects and methods were not necessarily comparable.) HIV-2, the virus variant found particularly in West Africa, appears to have a lower mother-child transmission rate. (*AIDS in the World* 1992:633–636) Where maternal health and health care are poor, transmission rates appear to be higher. (FitzSimons 1993:25–26)

A handful of documented cases that HIV can be passed on in breast-feeding have been queried by subsequent researchers (Panos 1990b:44), but they served as the basis for heated debates on whether HIV positive mothers should breast-feed. The poor, rural woman, who finds herself confronted with advice and warnings, is probably put in an impossible position. While a mother in Europe could resort to the elaborate paraphernalia which ensure safe bottle-feeding, the village mother might need to rely on unsafe water supplies, unsterilized equipment and expensive milk substitutes, which greatly increase the child's risk of both gastro-enteritis and malnutrition. In such circumstances, the World Health Organization recommends breast-feeding as the better alternative. (Panos 1990b:44–45; see criticism, Desclaux 1994)

A potentially far more politically charged debate is beginning to surface about the rights of HIV positive women to produce children at all. It centres on the issues of whether women have the right to give birth to 'doomed' babies, or to give birth when they themselves are 'doomed', and the baby will either die young or live to be a 'burden' on society once the mother, and usually the father, too, is dead. Even evidence which suggests that AZT, given to pregnant women, could reduce the number of paediatric transmissions, may be countered with the argument that this is simply producing healthy orphans.

With the exception of a small number of women in contemporary developed countries, the majority of the world's women appear to want to produce children. Since the future of any community depends on its physical need to reproduce itself, it is not surprising that the great majority of societies include strong pro-natalist themes in both secular and religious teachings; Genesis' injunction to 'be fruitful, and multiply, and replenish the earth', is widely incorporated in reproductive norms. Similarly the pity, the scorn or the ostracism which 'barren' women experience make them eager to fulfill the expectations of motherhood which marriage entails, not once, but usually repeatedly, and often at least until they produce a son. Many women in developed countries bear less than the 2.1 children necessary to replace population each generation, but in developing countries women continue to produce large numbers of children. In 1988, the women of China, notwithstanding its one-child population policy, produced on average 2.4 children, India 4.3 and Brazil 3.4. In much of sub-Saharan Africa, women had more than six with Nigeria averaging 7, Tanzania 7.1 and Kenya 8.1. (O'Connor 1991:47) The passage of bridewealth from husband's to wife's family often entails a contractual obligation for the woman – or a substitute provided by her family if she fails to fall pregnant – to produce a child. Childbirth often serves as a *rite de passage* into adulthood; a woman who does not produce may be in the same unenviable position as a man who never went through his society's mandatory male initiation process – a social failure. She risks being supplanted by a more fertile rival, particularly where polygyny is permitted. She will have no children to look after her in old age. When her husband dies he will have no legal heir; his land may revert to his family and she may have to leave the plot she cultivated. (The pronatalist theme may also mean that a woman, barren or fertile, is inherited by her dead husband's brother. In areas where HIV is prevalent, such leviratic marriages may expose both of them to new risks of infection.)

There is a growing tendency to counsel couples who are at risk of producing an HIV-positive child to practise contraception or abortion. Dr Marvellous Mhloyi of the University of Zimbabwe's sociology department, says that parents should be strongly advised to follow this advice. The risk of leaving orphaned children and of exposing older children to the additional trauma of losing a sibling to AIDS must be discussed. However, as he points out: 'These options are difficult within a cultural context where women derive status from maternity.' (1991:48)

The Savagery of Life: powerlessness and vulnerability

An aspect of the problem often overlooked is that men, especially men from poor and marginalized communities, may also derive status from paternity. To prove one's manhood by fathering a child is often a purely biological statement; where the father is himself hardly more than a child, there is little capacity to assume social and financial responsibility for the action. Nevertheless, it may give him personal affirmation of his virility and enhance his status with his peers.

Where fertility has so many complex social corollaries, the counsel against having children offered to HIV-infected people may be little short of a personal disaster. Positive HIV status is often discovered during pregnancy, or when a child fails to thrive. Where fertility is important, where the woman is economically dependent on her husband, or where she fears violence or desertion should her husband know her HIV status, she may keep the information to herself. She may go ahead with a pregnancy, hoping that her baby will be spared. Dr Janet Mitchell, an obstetrician at New York's Harlem Hospital, says the medical profession's surprise at such seemingly irrational responses stems from their failure to see such decisions from the women's point of view. Even a 50% risk may seem acceptable. (Panos 1990b:47) For women, childbearing may be seen as life affirming, a window into the future, a reason to live.

While the woman in the remote village may not know she is HIV positive, in the developed world there is a good chance she may find out before she falls pregnant or early enough in her pregnancy to have a safe abortion. Increasingly, such women are being encouraged not to produce children. Ronald Bayer questions the whole ethic of such preventive intervention: 'the reformist zeal that so frequently has attended efforts to save children from their parents' misdeeds may merge with the eugenic tradition of challenging the absolute right of parents

95

to bear children at high risk of congenital disorders.' (1991:193–194) He adds: 'That the women who are most at risk for bearing infected children are poor, black, and Hispanic, and most often intravenous drug users or their sexual partners, heightens the sense of disquiet about the prospect of a repressive turn in public policy.' (ibid.:194) Bayer argues that women are particularly vulnerable to the loss of their reproductive rights if it is believed to be in the public interest. He quotes, for instance, the 100,000 retarded women sterilized in the USA between 1920 and 1973 to prevent them transmitting their condition to their children. (ibid.:195) The gay demands for privacy, non-discrimination and non-repressive measures early on in the epidemic set a tolerant and voluntarist tone, but as the number of AIDS cases grows, policies could become more repressive.

Bayer writes that current counselling for couples with hereditary, genetic disorders essentially leaves the ultimate choice on child-bearing in their own hands. (ibid.:196–197) The feminist movement has added an explicitly political dimension, insisting on the woman's right to control her own body. 'The notion of choice has served as an ideological cornerstone of the political program of the movement for reproductive rights and women's health.' (N. Wikler quoted in Bayer 1991:199) Despite these developments, the poor or marginalized HIV-positive American woman is still likely to be advised against having a baby; some of the more strident critics of this approach have condemned it as 'a strategy for racial depopulation, as genocidal.' (ibid.:208)

Unlike other inherited diseases which may lead to the birth of a small number of disabled children each year, who will be dependent on parents or the State for care, AIDS is an epidemic, and a very costly one in every way. A child born to infected parents at worst will die in the first few months or years of life, at best will probably have to face life as an orphan. As in so many other areas, these hard facts are forcing even liberal thinkers to evaluate very carefully what constitutes appropriate HIV/AIDS counselling. AIDS has the unhappy knack of pitting 'individual rights' against 'public good'. In spotlighting the paediatric epidemic, policy guidelines carry a whiff of eugenics disquieting to those who are concerned with issues of individual reproductive choice.

Such choices tend to be the prerogative of a minority of the world's women. Most neither know what options there are, nor have the resources to select from them if they do. How do you reach a poor, isolated, illiterate rural or urban woman, who is not at school, at work or at church or a clinic attender? The AIDS epidemic has, if nothing else, produced some innovative solutions. In Port au Prince, for instance, the hundreds of brightly painted beauty parlours dotted throughout poor neighbourhoods provide information to Haitian women; the proprietors act as effective educators and condom distributors, reaching three-quarters of the city's women. (Panos 1990b:77) Elsewhere in the world, outreach programmes take the message to prostitutes, hawkers, commuters on buses and trains, people having lunch in the park. Musicians, drama groups, puppet-shows, videos, travel into dusty corners of the countryside with the AIDS message.

The message is only the first step. Armed with the facts, do women have the power, individually or as political pressure groups, to ensure they are allowed to practise safer sex?

Curiously, some of the more successful projects have been with women often seen as the most exploited and oppressed – prostitutes in developing countries. In Accra, Ghana, in 1987, a group of prostitutes were selected from a community to learn about condom use and act as educators and condom distributors. 'Two years later, clients who refused to use condoms faced a clear choice – they were told to wear

them or go away, since in the words of Alice, chairperson of a prostitutes' association, "we can't risk getting this disease just for money.'"
(Panos 1990b:82)

Similar projects in, for instance, Nigeria and Thailand have also given
the women some control. For such programmes to be successful it is
important for all the prostitutes in an area to agree to refuse a client
who will not use a condom. In negotiating this issue the prostitutes
themselves serve as educators for their often-uninformed clients.
Where women see sex as a purely cost-benefit exercise, it is easier for
them to make these demands; research projects often show that women
who use condoms with clients, do not use them with their regular
lovers. Another factor in successful programmes is the inclusion of
other health care services, or perhaps training in literacy, sewing or
other income generating activity which would make the women less
dependent on prostitution.

Such well-intended programmes may founder on hard political reality.
Prostitution is often part of a more complex web of socially disap-
proved, even criminal, behaviour, rather than simply a form of self-
employment. In such situations, attempts to empower women may
meet with resistance not only from clients, but pimps, bar-owners,
even local authorities who rely on the commercial sex industry.
Prostitutes in Madras, India report that 'most men do not use condoms
because they say it lessens sexual pleasure. The woman herself has no
power to demand its use as she is often uneducated, poor and dominated by the police-politician-pimp-nexus that controls the trade.'
(Panos 1990b:33)

In a report on Indonesian prostitution, *WorldAIDS* notes that as the first
HIV cases surfaced, and people called for brothels to be shut down, it
became clear that 'at all levels of the sex industry, military personnel

play a major role with pimps paying substantial bribes to officers, and brothels providing jobs and investment opportunities for all ranks. The civilian authorities, too, are heavily involved, and the urgent, if ineffective, response to the AIDS scare, reflected government officials' desire to protect their business interests.' (January 1993:12) Elsewhere, corrupt police, health officials who issue certificates stating women are HIV-free, travel agents offering sex tourism packages, or brutal entrepreneurs shipping young girls across borders into what amounts to sex slavery, are all part of an industry not calculated to roll back the AIDS pandemic.

Many of the world's prostitutes are not part of such an underworld. In parts of Europe, for instance, where prostitution is legalized and controlled, many women act on their own behalf, sometimes belong to their own unions, and can negotiate condom use with clients. Even those in less ideal circumstances may choose prostitution over the alternatives offered by well-meaning agencies, bent on re-training them. In New Guinea, where in many areas antagonistic sexual relationships have historically kept men and women in almost separate cultural camps, exchanging sex for services, gifts and money may not be seen as demeaning.

Reports suggest that 'for some women, the gradual commoditization of sex has meant rewards in terms of cash availability, freedom from traditional gender roles and enhanced self-esteem.' (*WorldAIDS* Sept 1993:2) A survey on prostitution in the Gambia challenges the view that women go into prostitution as the only alternative to destitution. In this area of West Africa, as in nineteenth-century France, prostitutes come from all sections and classes of society. Although some might prefer alternative occupations, many choose to remain in the profession. (Pickering, Todd *et al.* 1992)

Payment for sexual services often forms part of a complex set of survival strategies. In my own research in a black South African township, women who traded sex for trinkets, money or a roof over their heads, did not fall into an easily defined 'prostitute' category. They moved in and out of what might be termed 'the sex industry', depending on such factors as the availability of other work, their own needs for cash or accommodation, the arrival or absence of a partner, and the partner's maintenance payments. In a community where men were often regarded as unreliable – sexually, financially or emotionally – many women of all ages and classes deliberately chose not to marry, or even enter into long-term relationships. (van der Vliet 1991)

Our understanding of sexual relationships and gender inequality, particularly in developing countries, often suffers from Western bias and wholly inadequate research. They are notoriously difficult issues to study, but crucial to successful AIDS interventions. Programmes aimed at helping women negotiate condom use in all their relationships, short and long term, may be more useful than trying to divert them into more acceptable occupations or relationships.

Negotiating condom use is very complex, especially for a married woman, where it suggests she does not trust her husband, or that she herself is engaging in risky behaviour. Where producing children is a woman's expected role, condoms are particularly controversial. They are anyway an unpopular item in most places, and require male cooperation. For years, assumptions about male uncooperativeness and the female's lack of negotiating power, shaped the efforts of family planners. Some programmes, especially those where male sterilization was a significant option, did draw in men, but most were directed largely at women. Pro-natalist traditions meant women could not overtly influence family size, but often resorted either to those covert methods of abortion or infanticide which have always been under female control, or to modern methods of clandestine contraception such as the Pill, injection or IUD. Such methods are secret, and they do not require male cooperation. They empowered women, but without creating a culture of marital negotiation.

AIDS has overturned this strategy. If women wish to have men use condoms, negotiation and cooperation will be necessary. The 'female condom' does not change this situation; since it is hardly unobtrusive it cannot be under women's exclusive control. Sexual politics leaves women who want to avoid infection three options: stay out of the game, negotiate with men, or find a clandestine method of protection.

Anecdotal evidence suggests that some women, especially those who already have children, may opt for the celibacy option, but it seems an unlikely choice for most of the world's women.

The negotiation option is obviously the ideal, since it could have spill-over effects into other areas of decision-making such as family size, household budgeting, chore-sharing, and children's support. Evidence suggests that it may have limited effectiveness.

Many sociocultural variables, alone or in combination, can undermine a woman's potential to negotiate. Patriarchal relationships, machismo, pro-natalism, the availability of alternative women, the acceptance of multipartner relations and encouragement by peers, male control of critical resources like housing and land, the extreme youth of the woman, an anti-condom attitude among men, men's fear of loss of control over women, nonchalant attitudes to sexual abuse, even rape – each reflects the interrelationship of gender and power, and influences women's ability to control sex and reproduction. Even the suggestion that women may have the right to attempt such control, can elicit strong reaction. An article in the October 1994 edition of the news

The Politics of AIDS

magazine, *New African*, for instance, saw negotiation as a Western feminist abomination:

> The condom evangelists and safe sex missionaries seem especially preoccupied with changing men's behaviour. Their latest strategy has Western radical feminism written all over it. They want to turn African women under 25 into 'gatekeepers' who negotiate sexual relations and risk-reduction strategies. (p.17)

A worrying aspect of such attitudes is the anti-woman element surfacing in places experiencing heterosexual epidemics. As earlier chapters show, those caught up in the epidemic are very likely to look for someone to blame. All through history women have been useful scapegoats during epidemics. In 1438, when the plague struck Egypt, the Sultan's advisers believed it was God's punishment for 'fornication and blatant prostitution' (Dols 1977:114) and the Sultan prohibited all women from going out on the streets on pain of 'all kinds of maltreatment and even death.' (ibid.) Prostitutes have been the scapegoats during epidemics of cholera, gonorrhoea and syphilis in America and Europe. Even ordinary women can be blamed; today in Romania and Uganda HIV-infected women are categorized as prostitutes or 'loose' women. (Panos 1990b:49) In many places, even being in possession of a condom is enough to have a woman arrested on suspicion of prostitution. In Zimbabwe, parliamentarian Nathaniael Mutoko is reported to have declared in a debate: "If a pregnant woman is found to have AIDS she should be killed so that AIDS ends there, with her." (*The Argus* 9 March 1994) In Zaire, women, probably infected by their husbands, are blamed for the disease and sent home to their families, while the men find new women. (Panos 1990b:49) Schoepf *et al.* note: 'In a number of ... African countries, urban women, including prostitutes, traders, and others who escape male control, have been deported to rural areas.' (1988:217–218) They suggest that the conjunction of an economic crisis with the AIDS epidemic has made women a convenient focus of aggression. (ibid.)

If achieving negotiating power and control involves not only overcoming the disadvantages of poverty, illiteracy and isolation, but also somehow changing the myriad sociocultural impediments outlined above, women's empowerment looks to be a long way off. If it is to occur at all, it seems clear that the men will have to be brought on board. Unlike pregnancy, which was often ultimately the woman's responsibility, AIDS will affect the man, the woman and their children. Since men are the ones who control condom use, it is they who need to be given the message and convinced of its urgency. Informing their wives may be counter-productive; if a woman takes the message back to her husband, he might reject it as irrelevant, or uninformed, or even as an act of political control over her. Discussing sex at all is often impossible; women simply defer to men's wishes. To draw men into the AIDS strategy is going to require very situation-sensitive strategies.

Where women's empowerment strategies attempt to address other issues, such as males taking responsibility for caring for the AIDS sick, expect even further resistance. Currently the care of the sick and dying falls heavily on the women and girls, adding to their burdens; girls are often taken out of school for this task, or to take over farming once their mothers are too ill, entrenching the cycle of female disempowerment.

The third option – finding a clandestine method of protection – which women have resorted to in family planning, when male cooperation is not forthcoming – has the major disadvantage that at present there are no safe, female-controlled methods.

Why not? It was known from early on in the epidemic that substances such as nonoxynol-9, the basis of a contraceptive spermicide, might be useful. At tiny concentrations, one hundredth of that used on condoms, it 'quickly inactivates HIV and decreases the viability of HIV-infected lymphocytes *in vitro.*' (*AIDS in the World* 1992:402) Unfortunately, nonoxynol-9 (N-9) is detergent and can produce allergic reactions, and cervical or vaginal irritation in some women. It has also been shown to produce genital ulcers in some studies. Any such reaction could make women even more vulnerable to HIV. (Panos 1990b:30)

The few studies available are far from definitive. (Stone and Hitchcock 1994) For instance, some of the experimental research on HIV efficacy was carried out on prostitutes using sponges impregnated with N-9; one needs to ask whether the abnormal frequency of intercourse and the abrasive properties of the sponges under these conditions may have led to the problems. (ibid.:S287) N-9 has been in use in standard over-the-counter commercial spermicides for years. Package inserts and family planning literature warn that it may occasionally produce allergic reactions or irritation. Nevertheless, it is patently a relatively safe drug, and one would have assumed that research both to test its efficacy in different situations, and to develop other similar, woman-controlled products would have been a research priority.

Again the questions surface: was this line of research ignored because it was not as heroic as the quest for a vaccine? A humble microbicide used intra-vaginally in a gel, tablet or pessary form is not Nobel prize territory. Pharmaceutical companies, who are happy to create products, with often far-reaching side effects, which 'help' a patient, perhaps curing 40% or 80% or 100% of those who use it, may be wary of marketing a product that promises to prevent a condition as severe as AIDS. If it failed in even 5% of cases (and was cheap to boot) it could land manufacturers in great financial trouble. The fact that it was a 'woman's product' may also have given it less cachet, and created research 'blind spots'. Whatever the reasons, the literature has been almost silent on the issue of microbicides.

It was only at the IXth International Conference on AIDS in Berlin in 1993, that such chemical barriers went to the top of the agenda. Michael Merson, head of the WHO's Global Programme on AIDS told delegates: 'A vaginal microbicide, active against HIV and, ideally, against other STD pathogens too, could revolutionise AIDS prevention.' (*WorldAIDS* July 1993:4)

A selective microbicide which was not a spermicide would be particularly valuable. It would enable women to protect themselves against HIV yet become pregnant, making it acceptable, for instance, to the Roman Catholic Church. The search for new compounds is underway. Joep Lange, of the WHO's clinical research and drug development department says: "If we're honest about it, we're back to the beginning: if there had been one-tenth of the attention which was given to antiretrovirals for treatment, we'd be there already." (ibid.) It is little short of extraordinary that in an epidemic where it was realized from early on that women's powerlessness to negotiate condom use was a major risk factor, we have taken ten years to pay serious attention to the obvious alternative.

The factors that so affect women – poverty, illiteracy, social upheavals, family breakdowns, urbanization, mobility, changing social and sexual values – put the young at even greater risk, particularly where the vulnerability of youth is accompanied by the vulnerability of having a single mother.

James Grant, executive director of UNICEF writes: 'Most of the human faces of this epidemic are of children and youth. As many as two thirds of all HIV infections occur among young people before their 25th birthday. For young women in their teens, the rate of infection is twice to three times that of young men of the same age. And for those children born with an HIV infection, or orphaned through the loss of their parents to AIDS, childhood is far too short and far too painful.' (UNICEF 1993a:1)

Women suffer poor health care and health education, but often, through family planning or pregnancy, have some link into medical networks; many young people, especially in developing countries, have no contact with any health programmes at all, unless they become clinically ill. Malnutrition, parasites, infection go untreated. Health education and sex education are often minimal or absent in schools, and traditional sex education such as that offered in initiation schools, has fallen into disuse. For those who do not attend school, and where it is taboo to discuss sex with parents or older people, ignorance may be complete – or limited to what they can glean from equally uninformed peers. Even where information is available, many factors operate against knowledge translating into behaviour. Their vulnerability to HIV infection is sharpened by the nature of adolescence itself. Anthropologists Philip and Iona Mayer, commenting on theories of adolescence, suggest:

> It could be an ethological datum that human youth just 'are like that' – prone to play and display, to roaming and tussling, to exploring territorially and adventuring sexually. Alternatively, it could be a common response to a not uncommon social situation – the situation where a gerontocracy excludes youth more or less from 'real' public and domestic responsibilities, and also perhaps from adult sociable gatherings and recreation. (1970:181)

The Savagery of Life: powerlessness and vulnerability

Whether youth sub-cultures are a function of biological givens, or of the structure and power relations of society, it is certainly true that youth and maturity often inhabit separate worlds, with serious implications for inculcating ideas of safer sex.

While youth is a very varied phenomenon, the existence of youth sub-cultures, which are a law unto themselves, is well documented. Many traditional societies recognized this, and formally embodied two sets of rules – one for the young and another for adults; an abrupt break between them was created by an initiation rite, admitting youths to the adult world. For much of the rest of the world, especially in the cities, adolescence is spent in a culture of its own making. Whether this takes the form of slavish following of peer-group norms and fashions, and risk-taking, 'experimental' behaviour such as smoking, drinking or drug-taking, or the anti-social thrills of gang life, with its emphasis on violence and sex, it makes the messages that come from the parent generation at best questionable, at worst a challenge to the adolescent's new-found power, which must be defied. Just as sex became the centrepiece of gay liberation, so adolescents often use it as an instrument to express their rebellion and freedom. AIDS messages that do not take these underlying meanings into account will be unlikely to influence something as fundamental as adolescent sexual activity.

The problems are frequently compounded by the fact that the young do not see themselves as being at risk. For youth, death is for the old. Early warnings, unless they have personal experience of AIDS deaths in their peer group, often meet with disbelief and denial. A study of youths aged 14 to 18 in East and West Berlin, for instance, showed that 'even relatively well-informed and intelligent boys and girls in general do not feel that they are personally concerned [about HIV infection]. There seems to be a tendency to underestimate the danger and to rely on being able to trust the partner....' (Hessling and Heckmann (eds.) 1993:111) The flip-side of their belief in their own invulnerability may be a fatalistic acceptance of risk. A report on Tanzanian teenagers says some boys refer to contracting AIDS as *ajali kazini* – an occupational hazard. (*WorldAIDS* Nov 1993:4) A growing epidemic may serve to reinforce fatalism. As AIDS deaths continued to increase in Uganda, for instance, the use of condoms, which had gained acceptance among the youth in the late 1980s, declined; 'careless sexual behaviour resurfaced as individuals felt nothing was left that could be saved.' (*Southern Africa Political and Economic Monthly* June 1994:7)

In many developing countries, where population growth rates are high, the demographic pyramid has a very broad, youthful base. Since AIDS is a disease of the young, demographics alone ensure a large and growing pool of people vulnerable to infection.

This critical shift in demographic balance, which is a product of a fall in infant and childhood mortality, without a corresponding drop in birthrates, may aggravate the problem of adolescent conflict with adult values. The balance between older and younger members in a community could itself be a risk factor. AIDS researchers Aral and Holmes comment: 'When the number of young people is disproportionately large, they may also be less influenced by the social norms of the older generation. Consequently more of them may engage in behaviours that raise their STD risks. It is quite likely that the demographic shift has played a part in the epidemic of STDs and the increases in other phenomena of adolescence such as juvenile drug use and related crime.' (1991:23)

AIDS will skew the demographic pyramid further. The slow gains in infant survival rates of the last two decades in many areas of the developing world, will be reversed as paediatric transmission increases.

Women, who tend to become infected at a younger age than men, will die younger, but also produce less children. Deaths among young adults will accelerate. While lower birth rates, and deaths among infants and young children statistically offset deaths of adults to some extent, preventing a huge rise in the dependency ratio – the ratio of productive to non-productive population – the AIDS process in individual families is devastating.

In developing countries, where life expectancy is low, children have often been confronted with the loss of a parent in the prime of life. AIDS has added a traumatic twist to this tragedy; in its long slow course, it inevitably takes both parents, and perhaps siblings as well. The old safety-net of the extended family comes under increasing strain. In badly affected areas, a woman's co-wives and children, sisters- and brothers-in-law and their children may all be infected. With the whole network gone, children either have to look after one another, or depend on grandparents barely able to care for themselves.

The population, skewed by AIDS deaths, will have a disproportionate number of 5 to 15 year olds and elderly people. For the young, education and training could be forfeited to the demands of survival. Those elderly who lose their entire younger generation face the prospect of becoming 'geriatric orphans'.

Alan Fleming, looking at tropical African trends, notes that 'by the fiftieth year of the epidemic, if there is no control, society will be dominated numerically by 33% of the population being aged between 15 and 25 years and there will be only 15% aged more than 25 years, as compared to about 30% at present. Relative to the total population, there will be only half the expected skill and professional competence.' (1993:308) He argues that the shortage of older adults, both as producers and teachers, could force the young into being providers – in subsistence farming or in poorly paid jobs – to their own and their country's detriment. (ibid.)

Whether or not the epidemic retains its ferocity long-term, the problem of AIDS orphans is already serious. By 1993, the United Nations Children's Fund, UNICEF, estimated there were two million AIDS orphans, 90 per cent of them in sub-Saharan Africa. (UNICEF 1993:9) The WHO estimates the number will grow to between 10 and 15 million worldwide by 2000. (*WorldAIDS* March 1993:5) Even where there are family members living nearby, such children may face rejection because of the fear and stigma of AIDS. For such children, orphanages or a life on the streets are usually the only options. The trauma of family loss, rejection and financial and emotional insecurity add up to an unpromising start to a young life, reproducing poorly socialized, inadequately educated and vulnerable citizens. 'The savage irony of HIV is that its effects intensify the socioeconomic conditions in which it is most easily transmitted.' (*AIDS in the World* 1992:672)

Most powerless and vulnerable of all is the growing army of street children. Today estimated at 100 million, their numbers are destined to grow by leaps and bounds as societies can no longer absorb their AIDS orphans, and the young take to the streets where they live by their wits. Petty crime, prostitution and drug use create children inured to risk, and resistant to the 'safer sex' message. For street kids, sex has many meanings – money, comfort, status – and even where they know about AIDS they commonly disregard its message.

The overwhelming majority of street children are found in the cities of the developing world. Bombay, Nairobi, Rio de Janeiro, Johannesburg, Manila have large brigades of such children. Perhaps up to 80% have families; they return home at intervals, perhaps nightly, with their earnings, and are important contributors to the family income. The rest are street children proper, with no other real home. *WorldAIDS* describes their plight as one of 'constant struggle. Many earn a miserable living selling gum or cigarettes, shining shoes, washing cars or doing odd labouring jobs. Others scavenge on rubbish tips, deal drugs, or sell their bodies – sometimes just for a meal or a bed for the night.' (January 1994:7)

Ana Filgueiras, of the Brazilian Centre for the Defence of the Rights of Adolescents, paints a picture of the life of street children in Rio de Janeiro that makes it clear why such children are at great risk in the AIDS epidemic. She describes a brutal world where children cling together for protection. Early sexual intimacy is 'part of a broader atmosphere of immediate gratification when no one knows what is going to happen the next minute and where children want things to be done and desires to be filled right away.' (1992/3:22) Impatience, aggression, low self-esteem and self-destructive tendencies make cautious safe sex messages difficult to put across, particularly where sex itself is an important organizing principle. Filgueiras points out:

> Sex with several partners is a current norm, mostly for males. Further along this line, male power within the group is frequently based on the concept of masculinity which is itself based to a large degree on the level of sexual activity of the individual. This way, the male on the street can boost his social position and power within his group by maintaining multiple partners, either male or female. (1992/3:23)

Girls on the street in a macho society are particularly vulnerable, both to their peers and to sexual abuse by outsiders. Filgueiras accepts that for many, returning to impoverished and abusive homes is not an alternative; she outlines a long wish-list to help the Rio children – everything from safe shelters to legal aid, hotlines and mobile help

111

units. She urges government agencies to assume their responsibilities for providing for the children (1992/3:24), but as in so many places, the demands of street children must compete with countless others on the state. A particularly ominous note in Brazil, and elsewhere in Latin America, is the reported operation of death squads, which periodically 'clean the streets' of street children, often with popular support.

> In Brazil, hundreds of children are killed each year by squads of off-duty military police and self-appointed vigilantes; in Guatemala, uniformed police and private security firms have beaten, tortured and killed streetchildren. (*WorldAIDS* January 1994:8–9)

Without secure homes and jobs, children and youths often find themselves on the bottom rung of the underworld ladder; they are exploited by older drug dealers, crime syndicates, pimps, even corrupt police. According to Peter Dalglish, of Street Kids International, 'in many countries, members of the police basically use streetkids as another source of revenue, extorting money from them and ill-treating them.' (*WorldAIDS* January 1994:9)

In lives of such fear and misery, the chance that they might fall victim to AIDS five or ten years from now must seem hardly worth considering. Hounded and abused by mainstream society, such children are hardly likely to believe its messages; they could be forgiven for believing that society may regard AIDS an ally in its attempts to 'clean the streets'.

Some street children, particularly in Asian countries with high levels of injecting drug use, are at risk of HIV from infected needles, but for most the threat is from sexual relationships. Not only street children, but all children from impoverished, abusive or negligent homes may be driven into early sexual relationships, whether for money or comfort. All of them are at particular risk. Girls who are not yet physically completely mature are more prone to injury during sex, and so to HIV infection. Early pregnancy, back-street abortion and unsafe blood transfusions add to their risks. For young boys, homosexual sex with adults is especially risky. For boys, too, the available condoms are often too big and manufacturers seem unwilling to produce child-size varieties. (*WorldAIDS* January 1994:9)

Children may also become bait for the lucrative sex tourism industry. Such tourists in, for instance, Thailand, Sri Lanka, and the Philippines are lured with brochures emphasizing 'the youth, beauty and compliance of their people... Promotional material is usually sexually explicit and aimed at both heterosexual and homosexual tourists.' (*WorldAIDS* March 1992:6) Many of these tourists (and home-grown clients) are demanding younger and younger sexual partners, in the belief that they are less likely to be infected with HIV. Governments are faced with a dilemma: while acknowledging that the alarming growth in infections poses enormous problems down the track, tourism is a major contributor of hard currency, and provides 'employment' for many unemployed women and children. Even where governments have clamped down, economic reality may frustrate their efforts. In the Philippines, for instance, after the overthrow of the Marcos regime, citizens and government joined forces to eradicate child prostitution. Police and immigration authorities raided and closed down brothels which had offered children to paedophiles, and deported foreigners found patronizing them. For the children and their families who depended on this trade, business simply moved elsewhere. (ibid.)

While governments may act to protect, educate or care for the young, the young themselves usually have little power to influence the policies devised for them. Often cultural taboos on, for instance, sex education, condoms for children, or STD clinics where the young can be treated in privacy, leave gaps in whatever programmes are available. Politicians may not be willing to risk instituting such controversial programmes.

Where children have been sucked into the political process and become the footsoldiers of political conflicts, the safer sex message may be particularly hard to instil. Christine Obbo writes of Uganda, for instance: 'During the 1970s, many children in both rural and urban areas rebelled against parental and school authorities as the general atmosphere of societal anarchy and state terrorism made life uncertain and violence looked glamorous.' (Obbo 1993:8) In South Africa, the 1970s saw the politicization of large segments of black youth. Schools became political forums, bastions of resistance against the apartheid system, and the children became an army, militant and beyond the control of adults.

racial predujice

The war against apartheid has been won, but the years of 'ungovernability', which characterized their struggle, has made many of this generation of South African youth volatile; politicians will tread warily in their dealings with them. Messages of caution and moderation will not necessarily find a receptive audience. For some children, angry at being robbed of their childhood, the realization that change has not translated into immediate material benefits, may leave them rebellious. 'They feel abandoned by those whom they looked up to and who are now part of the authority structures which appear to act impersonally.' (Ramphele 1994:39; see also Everatt and Milner 1994; Straker 1992)

The young, and particularly young women, face a formidable array of hurdles in their quest for the control over their lives which would help them avoid AIDS. Despite the problems, carefully targeted interventions can motivate behavioural change – or at least ensure the acceptability of information. Programmes that emphasize peer group education; outreach projects focused on youth venues that have credibility, and preferably ongoing communication, with their target group, such as school nurses, youth clubs, discos and social gathering areas; campaigns associated with youth role models such as pop stars, athletes and movie stars; and information sessions addressed by young HIV-positive people help overcome resistance to 'adult' messages. Hard-to-reach street children have been targeted with a video cartoon and comic book, *Karate Kids*, based on the street leader hero, Karate, who with his girlfriend Rosa, launches a campaign to teach children about AIDS after one of their number is infected and dies. It provides explicit AIDS information, and is now translated into 14 languages and used in 100 countries. The storyline incorporates the common experiences of the world's street children and was pre-tested on children in Nairobi, Colombo, Manila, Rio de Janeiro, New York City and Toronto, and children's feedback was used to modify the material. Whether the project will succeed long term is still unknown, but it certainly stimulates discussion of sexual health, street life and AIDS. Predictably, it has also provoked strong criticism from those in authority, uncomfortable with its explicit style. (*AIDS in the World* 1992:360–361)

The resistance of adults to empowering the young, whether by educating them in lifeskills or sexuality, providing them with condoms, or involving them in policy-making, is an issue of adult politics, part of the games adults play, in this case often to the detriment of their children. *In AIDS: the Second Decade – A Focus on Youth and Women,* UNICEF concludes its assessment of the underlying societal conditions which fuel the AIDS pandemic with these words:

No programme, no amount of money, no support will make a difference if it does not provide youth and women with the means to control their lives. They must know that society will back their right to self-determination. Their strength is the societal tool that will contain the spread of AIDS. (1993a:30)

The question is whether the political realities of governments, gender and generation will allow them such empowerment.

CHAPTER 5

LESSONS FROM THE AIDS PANDEMIC

No disease in history has raised such complex issues, required such a wide range of responses, or so mercilessly unveiled the pre-existing serious imbalances, inadequacies and inequities embedded in health and social systems around the world.
Charles Cameron (in *AIDS in the World* 1992:449)

Although AIDS is a new addition to the catalogue of human misery, it provides, as health economist Charles Cameron suggests, a potent lens through which to view the human condition. In this book, I have explored the social dimensions of the pandemic, and particularly the way it reflects prevailing relations of power and powerlessness. I have also looked at explanations of who gets AIDS and why, as products of macro- and micropolitical processes. Coping with the pandemic, and turning it around, is going to involve changing these power relationships and political processes, or finding ways around them for individuals or groups. Those who are

117

trapped into powerlessness are sitting ducks in areas where seroprevalence is high.

Becoming infected with HIV is not a random medical event. More perhaps than any other major health threat, it demonstrates the extent to which disease is in fact embedded in the social, political, economic, cultural, behavioural and medical experience of individuals. Understanding AIDS requires that we understand what Guenter Risse has called the 'ecology' of disease – 'the dynamic relationships between the biosocial environment and humans.' (1988:33) The issues, as they have emerged in this book, are complex; if we are to avoid simplistic explanations and strategies, the disease must be seen in this ecological context. I believe it is helpful to try to represent this context schematically, dividing the field of causality into biomedical, social and behavioural areas. (Fig.1)

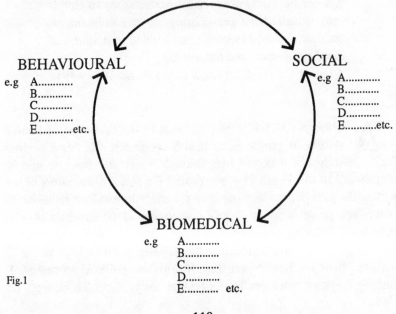

BEHAVIOURAL

e.g   A............
      B............
      C............
      D............
      E............etc.

SOCIAL

e.g A............
    B............
    C............
    D............
    E............etc.

BIOMEDICAL

e.g   A............
      B............
      C............
      D............
      E............ etc.

Fig.1

Although the factors do not necessarily always fit neatly into one or the other area – for instance, is 'substance abuse' actually a biomedical problem, a social pathology or an individual behavioural aberration? – the merit of trying to schematize causation in this way is that it reveals the interaction of causes. The risk of an epidemic in any society or community will depend on the levels of risk in these interacting factors.

For instance, if a number of the social factors, which we believe operate to precipitate an epidemic, were in place – poverty, gender inequality, many street children, low levels of education – but multipartner sexual relations, STDs and HIV seroprevalence were low, in a society with strong religious controls on sexual behaviour, the epidemic would grow slowly if at all. In a community where high levels of multipartner sex, substance abuse, condom resistance and risk-taking behaviour occur in a situation where HIV seroprevalence is high, affluence and a high standard of education will not protect its members from exposure.

Such a model of causation also protects us from falling into the trap of mono-causal explanations – and consequent reliance on simplistic solutions. For instance, the knee-jerk reaction against prostitutes as the cause of the epidemic could be avoided if we saw their activities not only in the light of the social factors which lead to their reliance on commercial sex, but also of the behavioural and cultural factors which make such sex possible, and the biomedical factors of STDs, health care and HIV seroprevalence which make it risky. If prostitution is seen in its context, it becomes clear that it will not be eliminated by police swoops on brothels, however appealing this 'solution' might be to ambitious politicians or church leaders.

The model also enables us to see where realistic interventions are possible. In the example of prostitution, the idealists might say that we must eliminate poverty and the exploitation of women, but, in the short run, better health care, especially the elimination of other STDs, adequate supplies of condoms, and support groups which enable prostitutes to negotiate condom use, are more pragmatic interventions.

There is, of course, a great appeal in the quest for 'the grand solution', be it biomedical (a vaccine which prevents infection or a drug that cures it), social (the elimination of poverty, war, labour migration, exploitation, oppression, irrationality and greed, from the human condition), or behavioural (chastity before marriage and fidelity thereafter, and the elimination of injectable drugs, and those substances which would undo the chastity/fidelity package).

We have seen that biomedical 'magic bullets' are still a long way off. More discouraging is the fact that even where medical science has provided us with highly effective solutions – vaccines for measles and hepatitis B, or effective drugs for TB or STDs, for instance – social and behavioural factors may make them unavailable, or ill-utilized, in a particular situation. The danger that HIV vaccines or cures may be beyond the financial reach of the countries most affected, is very real, just as we see them using untested blood, even in situations where poverty forces those most at risk to sell their blood for money. In fact, medical technology has already provided us with a very effective protection against HIV – the condom – but social and behavioural factors undermine its usefulness.

Social solutions win all-round applause for good intentions and political correctness, but they offer little hope in the short term. Similar solutions have been offered for problems as varied as rapid population growth, tuberculosis, poverty, crime and drug abuse, but without any notable general success. If the last three decades have not changed the world economic order, or the plight of developing countries, or the lot of the United States' underclass, it is unlikely that the AIDS epidemic will produce the necessary miracle. In fact, as discussed earlier, it may lead the rich to despair of, and abandon, the poor. It is also not certain that improved social circumstances would automatically reverse a growing epidemic. Unless the newly-contented followed the behavioural codes of safer sex, improved social conditions would not necessarily protect them; if the virus were still abroad, the epidemic could merely move upmarket.

Behavioural change focused on safer sex strategies seems at present to hold the most promise of success. In its extreme form – premarital chastity and marital fidelity – it is a prescription with a universally less-than-satisfactory track-record. If even the threat of hell-fire, which some of its advocates have preached, were not enough to ensure obedience, the fear of AIDS will probably not bring compliance either. More realistic versions of the safer sex message have met with some success, demonstrating that in certain circumstances, the message is saleable. If everybody could be persuaded to heed it, the pandemic would be stopped in its tracks. However, individual behaviour is itself dependent on social factors such as gender inequalities and cultural norms like machismo or pro-natalism, and on biomedical factors such as condom availability and health services, which facilitate or retard behavioural change. Whatever the obstacles, strategies must target the individual, since it is the individual who provides the crucial interface between good ideas and epidemic control. Properly informed and supported, individuals can find ingenious ways around social and medical barriers. American gays challenging FDA procedures, Ghanaian prostitutes banding together to deny clients sex without condoms, Zambian schoolboys setting up anti-AIDS clubs with members pledged to chastity before marriage, Ugandan Boy Scouts working for AIDS awareness badges, US high school students organizing AIDS telephone hotlines, and myriad peer group education initiatives, all speak to the innovativeness of individuals under threat.

Each of the 'grand solutions' has its proponents, most of whom genuinely believe that such a solution is possible, and they are willing to work hard and long to achieve it. However there is a danger, as we have seen in the course of this book, that espousing grand solutions sometimes conceals a political agenda. Blaming the disease on foreigners, prostitutes or urban women, or more broadly on poverty and under-development, and offering to deal with such problems, provides useful handholds in a political career. Insisting that AIDS is the wages of sin and that only those who follow a specific religious or political agenda will be saved, or that it reflects the destruction of family values which your dispensation will restore, may also serve to guide the public into your political or ideological camp.

Espousing one of these solutions may force its champions to discount other factors in the ecology of the epidemic. Randall Packard, for instance, in a paper on AIDS in Africa, questions behavioural models of the epidemic – what he refers to as 'the central paradigm of heterosexual transmission' (1989:3) – with its focus on 'sexual promiscuity.' (ibid.) He believes the question ought to have been: 'What is the social context within which HIV transmission occurs in Africa?' (ibid.:5) This is, of course, a valid question but it does not deliver a short-term solution. If one settles for explanations at the level of social context, one is also forced to seek solutions at this level. If AIDS is a result of 'exploitive', capitalist production which has led to 'semi-proletarianized', impoverished communities, (ibid.:7) what strategies are appropriate to turn the tide? Packard concludes:

Before we waste millions on the type of behaviour modification model of intervention now being explored, we must have a higher degree of certainty about how HIV is being transmitted and what the real risk factors are, as well as knowledge of the social and economic context within which risk factors are set. If the primary risk factor is being poor and unemployed, then our proposed interventions must address the causes of this condition. We must not allow AIDS to become one more symptom for which the West finds a cure without addressing the underlying causes of this and many other health problems.' (ibid.:19)

The danger of this analysis is the impossibility of realizing the solution Packard recommends in time to stem the AIDS epidemic. While behaviour may be amenable to short-term interventions, social change is a long-term affair. To limit your strategy to the social and economic context is to deprive people of control over their lives. Like blaming victims, blaming systems achieves little. It is ultimately a profoundly disempowering analysis.

An end to poverty and struggle are goals to be pursued vigorously; a successful strategy to deal with the immediate epidemic would be part of such goals. An uncontrolled AIDS epidemic, on the other hand, could set back Africa's cause by decades.

As the epidemic has progressed, it has become increasingly clear that individual behaviour is 'the ultimate determinant of vulnerability.... A thorough examination of individual behaviours that expose people to HIV infection, including the community and larger societal dimensions of these behaviours, leads to a central conclusion: personal empowerment is the antithesis of vulnerability.' (*AIDS in the World* 1992:578–579)

Failing 'grand solutions', how can we effect this personal empowerment? If we examine the causality model presented above, at what points on the circle are interventions possible, particularly in the short term? Are such interventions contra-indicated by factors at work elsewhere in the model? Given that we have a growing pandemic and shrinking funds, are there cost-effective ways to intervene?

Information, despite the problems in translating knowledge into behaviour, remains the *sine qua non* of individual empowerment; until individuals have a clear, complete, unvarnished picture of the disease, and how it can be avoided, appropriate behaviour modification is impossible. At the same time, the myriad complex tactics which enable individuals to use the information, and which this book has described, must be implemented. AIDS education is an on-going process, not an event. It is not a matter of putting up a poster or giving a lecture. It must happen in a context which supports the individual's efforts. Provided the political will and support is there, many of these programmes can be devolved to organizations such as churches, trade unions, youth groups and other non-governmental organizations where better targeted campaigns are possible.

The most cost-effective projects are probably those which rely on specific biomedical interventions: safe blood supplies; vigorous control of STDs which facilitate HIV transmission; sterile medical equipment; sterile syringes and needles, whether for medical purposes or injecting drug users, available without prescription at pharmacies or through needle exchange programmes; the avoidance of unnecessary invasive medical procedures; adequate supplies of reliable, affordable condoms wherever those at risk may be, including controversial locations like schools and prisons; confidential HIV counselling and testing for those who require it; the expansion of existing medical facilities such as well-baby and antenatal clinics to incorporate HIV services.

A further spin-off from these interventions would be their positive effects on other health conditions such as STDs, and the spread of hepatitis B, currently carried by hundreds of millions of people around the world. (Aral and Holmes 1991:22)

All these suggestions might look elementary; the shocking truth is that in many of the countries where AIDS is on the rampage, such simple measures are beyond the reach of the national budget. Diverting some of the billions of dollars, currently being spent on AIDS in the developed world, to these purposes – or finding additional funds – might be the most cost-effective intervention currently available. At the IXth International Conference on AIDS, in Berlin in June 1993, Michael Merson informed delegates that "by tailoring educational campaigns to local communities, distributing condoms and clean needles, and treating the sexually transmitted diseases that foster the spread of HIV, health agencies could cut the rate of new infections by half throughout the developing world." (*Newsweek* June 21 1993:49) Even the United States has spent relatively little on STDs and, in the view of the *Newsweek* report, effectively encourages the sharing of needles among drug users in the more than 40 states where needles are treated as contraband. (ibid.)

In the complex social and behavioural context of the pandemic, short of a vaccine or cure, the medical breakthrough which would probably make the most dramatic contribution to slowing down the spread of HIV, would be a woman-controlled virucide. The extreme vulnerability of women in the face of the disease at present would be substantially reduced, and the disastrous domino effect of orphaned children and paediatric AIDS would be averted. Such a virucide would probably protect both partners, but men would still be able to protect themselves as well, if they wished, and the more difficult and problematic issues of what Uganda called 'zero-grazing' – chastity or fidelity – could be left to individuals and couples to resolve.

Such a medical breakthrough would probably not escape the mesh of societal factors. Control over the resource and its distribution would doubtless be entwined in politics, religion, economics, morality, ethics, law, just as everything to do with this epidemic appears to be, but it would perhaps present less insoluble problems than other strategies, especially given the urgency of the issue, and particularly from the woman's perspective.

If AIDS has done nothing else, it has forced people to rethink their positions on every issue touched by the pandemic, from sex, death and disease to mother's milk. Sclerotic laws and conventions about condoms and needles, prostitutes and homosexuality, drug-testing and commercial blood donation, the safety and necessity of medical procedures, patients' rights to information, euthanasia, sex education in schools, prisoners' rights, reproductive rights, media's responsibilities, the role of disease 'activists' and medical confidentiality, to name but a few, have all been put to the test by the pandemic. The results of such scrutiny may well bear fruit for a whole range of related problems, such as faster and more efficient drug testing procedures, activist programmes for a range of other diseases, including informing patients about their rights and alternatives, and more pragmatic approaches to health education issues. The inadequacies of expensive tertiary medical care, and of national health care policies, have also spotlighted the need for increasing emphasis on primary health care, and alternatives to hospital care, in community-based hospices, or via assistance to people caring for patients at home. Reactivating – and supporting – existing or traditional coping mechanisms, such as home care and the 'buddy' system developed in gay communities, may be a lot more useful than yet more heroic attempts to reinvent the wheel by outsiders. AIDS may lead us to some creative thinking on the provision of primary health care among the urban poor, but especially for the invisible poorest – the rural people who lie on the fringes of even rudimentary charity-driven church and 'good works' clinics, but not beyond the reach of HIV.

At its best the pandemic has created a global network of researchers and medical professionals locked onto the AIDS problem with terrier-like ferocity. It has provided a challenge and a goal of enormous dimensions, and has, as Robert Gallo writes, the capacity to 'force openness and collaboration in science among nations.' (1991:221) AIDS research has generated new insights into the nature of infectious diseases, neurological conditions, and a range of AIDS-related cancers which will in turn benefit other areas of medical research. 'Vaccine research, research on basic virology, immunology, and molecular biology have already been greatly enhanced by AIDS research. So has antiviral chemotherapy.' (Gallo 1991:232) At its worst, of course, AIDS has the capacity to precipitate the kind of destructive, internecine politico-scientific warfare that dogged Gallo's own laboratories for years.

In the criticisms levelled at the lavish spending on AIDS, we tend to forget at times that science is a seamless web. Just as seemingly grandiose space programmes yielded information and technology which have penetrated everywhere from medicine and ecology, to computer games and improved cooking utensils, so, in searching for the key to AIDS, we may unlock the door to cures for many other conditions.

For all that it may advance medical frontiers, for the present AIDS has caused much alarm and despondency in the medical profession. It has been a baptism by fire for the generation of doctors who trained in the post-polio period and, particularly in Western countries, have never had to face an epidemic for which they had no cure. It has been a humbling and, for some, a terrifying experience. Doctors, by the nature of their work, always confront disease and death at close quarters, but the age of antibiotics had largely liberated them from the fear of working with their patients. Even potentially lethal hepatitis B infection could be countered with a barrage of medical weaponry – and the same safety procedures as they will now need to protect themselves from HIV! AIDS has left them personally and professionally vulnerable. From being a profession which could cope with most of the conditions it encountered, short of the chronic degenerative diseases of the elderly, it was suddenly faced with growing numbers of young, hopeless cases for which even palliative treatments were initially unavailable. Confronting a mounting death toll among people in the prime of life, was something they had not been trained for. 'People so young are not supposed to die. These deaths challenged the ideology of the coming-if-not-quite-arrived triumph of modern medical science implicitly provided to young doctors in medical education.' (Bosk and Frader 1991:163)

AIDS took its toll on the profession. Like those involved in the care of other terminal diseases, many experienced burnout. Some simply refused to work with AIDS patients, either directly, or by choosing geographic locations or fields of medicine which limited their exposure to infected people. Bosk and Frader write of their experience in one American medical school, where policy prohibited students from refusing to care for HIV-infected patients. Students were angry that the policy had been formulated without consulting them; had they been aware of it before entering, they might have chosen another school. 'Doctors, they believe, should have as much freedom as lawyers, accountants, executives, or others to accept or reject 'clients' or 'customers'.' (1991:159)

There is nothing new in doctors avoiding or evading certain categories of patient. From the less-than-heroic flight of the medieval plague doctors, and of those in Philadelphia's yellow fever outbreak in 1793 (Fox 1988:90) to the refusal of some hospitals in nineteenth-century America to accommodate STD cases, history is full of examples of just such reactions. (Brandt 1987:43–45) Bosk and Frader believe that, in the case of AIDS, it is the unique combination of circumstances surrounding the epidemic which accounts for doctors' negative behaviour: 'changing tolerances of risk, the shift to an occupation bounded by entrepreneurial rules rather than professional duties, a specific fear of the terrible outcome should one acquire AIDS from a patient, objections to some of the specific behaviour that lead to AIDS, and class and racial bias.' (1991:163)

Whatever their aversion to the disease or its sufferers may be, the majority of doctors worldwide seem not to have refused to treat AIDS patients. Even if they believe that a particular case of HIV infection is the result of behaviour over which the individual could have had control, it does not exclude the 'guilty' individual from treatment. In fact, current explanatory models of many diseases 'blame' the sufferer; smoking, incorrect eating, insufficient exercise, excessive alcohol consumption, recreational drugs – somewhat equivalent to the 'dirt', 'gluttony', and intemperance of nineteenth-century explanations (Rosenberg 1988:19) – all lie within the individual's control. None of the victims of such habits is turned away by medicine, although unrepentant smokers are beginning to risk the refusal of expensive therapeutic procedures.

What should be done when contemporary doctors do refuse to treat HIV/AIDS patients? Looking at the problem in historical perspective, Daniel Fox suggests that ultimately the question may be answered by negotiating the terms on which doctors would be willing to treat them; as in the past 'epidemics offered physicians opportunities as well as risks.' (1988:87) Fox believes 'a new cadre of plague doctors now

129

serve in dedicated AIDS units or treat most of the persons with AIDS in particular hospitals. Their rewards are often access to research funds or academic status rather than income alone.' Fox sees a continuity between Chaucer's physician who delighted in the 'gold he kept from pestilence', and the well-known academic physician who said in Fox's presence, "AIDS has been good to me." (ibid.:94)

While some doctors may indeed become more powerful and control more resources as a result of AIDS, the glitter of modern medicine has been tarnished by the epidemic. The power of the medical profession has, as Charles Rosenberg points out, 'long been an object of reformist concern.' (1988:13) Western doctors are, of course, not alone in wielding influence; healers universally have an aura of authority, and often sacredness, intrinsic to their role. Although Western doctors have, by virtue of their expertise, often been central in policy-making surrounding disease, they have been rewarded with 'both power and resentment.' (Rosenberg 1988:17)

The 'confident belief in the unambiguous benefits of scientific medicine' which characterized the 1930s and 1940s had already begun to dissipate by the 1970s. (ibid.:16) AIDS was a body blow to that faith, and a warning that disease could only be fully understood and dealt with within a social and behavioural context. The insistence by gay activists, and later pressure groups such as infected haemophiliacs, that they were entitled not only to information and care, but that they had the right to influence policies that would affect them on everything ranging from confidentiality, to drug testing, to euthanasia, constituted a concerted attack on medical and health-policy conventions. Health workers, trained to instruct their patients, suddenly found their authority and knowledge challenged. The 'experts' were being questioned not only because they had failed to provide a quick fix for AIDS, but because faith in experts generally was eroding. Crises such as thalidomide, Three Mile Island, Chernobyl had all played their part. (Brandt 1987:200) The 'progress' of the technological age had left the world with holes in the ozone layer, acid rain and looming environmental degradation of frightening dimensions.

AIDS is part of this future vision, a future over which the experts are perceived to have lost control. In this environment, 'counter-experts' have emerged, who like those involved in the *Sunday Times* debate discussed earlier, may even question whether HIV is actually the cause of AIDS. They may endanger the whole programme of AIDS education in certain areas; as Robert Gallo warns, they also diminish the confidence in science and scientists, medicine, physicians and health care workers. He points out 'Undermining confidence in the only people working on AIDS is not likely to help unify our efforts to conquer it. Instead, it breeds distrust and perhaps frank hostility, often turning researchers into convenient targets for those whose business it is to attack government institutions and people.' (Gallo 1991:297) Whether we share Gallo's misgivings or not, AIDS has certainly played a part in initiating a new, if uneasy, balance between the 'powerful' expert and the 'powerless' public. What its role will be among healers in non-Western societies remains to be seen.

One side-effect of the doctors' relative impotence in the epidemic has been the growing role of nurses reported in some American studies. As doctors and technology provided solutions to medical problems in the antibiotic era, the nurse had come to be seen increasingly as the servant of the doctor, rather than a powerful health care expert in her (or less commonly, his) own right. Nursing patients through health crises sounded old-fashioned in situations where machines monitored every heartbeat and powerful drugs dripped into veins in carefully calibrated doses. In a study of the American nursing profession's response to AIDS, Fox, Aiken and Messikomer write that despite the

131

enormous stress of dealing with young people dying of a cruel and incurable disease, nurses are not, as had been feared, shying away from AIDS patients; many have chosen to work in specialized AIDS units or volunteer-and community-based units. For some, AIDS provides a chance to exercise again 'the entire range of physical, psychological, social, and spiritual interventions that nurses are characteristically, and, in many respects, singularly educated to provide.' (1991:130) AIDS is a disease of caring not curing, pre-eminently a field for nurses, rather than doctors and machines. Whether there will be any generalized and sustained re-evaluation of the nurse in the health care team as a result of the AIDS experience remains to be seen, but as a new generation of microbes begins their assault, nurses may again find themselves in the front line of patient care. Perhaps they will cease to be undervalued, largely mute and invisible in health care practice and policy.

Throughout this book we have examined the AIDS pandemic in relation to power and powerlessness – that vulnerability stems from lacking the power to control one's circumstances, that the power to affect the outcome of the epidemic is intimately tied into the social, political, economic and cultural purposes of those in control. Relations of power will direct the course of the pandemic, and in turn be transformed by it. In evaluating the response to AIDS in the world's industrialized democracies, David Kirp and Ronald Bayer conclude that

the politics of AIDS is the politics of democracy in the face of a critical challenge to communal well-being. The responses tell us a great deal not only about our recent past but also about how the next out-of-the-ordinary challenge to communal health is likely to be faced. If AIDS has taught us anything, it is that we can no longer believe that we are secure against such a threat. (*AIDS in the World* 1992:281)

That a minute virus could so up-end the grand design and certitudes of humankind is humbling, to say the least. It also points to a balance of power people seldom stop to consider – that between man and microbe. Our emergence and current ascendancy in the world is, in the earth's time-frame, a very recent phenomenon. Our arrogance in assuming humanity's continued dominion is also relatively recent. For hundreds of thousands of years we must assume that our forebears, like many people in today's small-scale societies, lived with due awareness of their precarious grasp on life, and their modest place in the blueprint of living things.

Microbes have been around since the beginning. Constantly mutating, they are admirably suited to life's changing circumstances. Our temporary triumph over them in the era of antibiotics would not even register as a blip on their evolutionary radar screen. Already, where they have been most exposed to the weapons we flaunt, in places like hospitals, they have chiselled away at our defences and created stubborn strains that defy our efforts to control them. Unsupervised treatment programmes, and street-peddling of powerful drugs in developing countries add to the problems. The more we throw at them the more practised they become at dodging, at creating new forms we cannot destroy – drug-resistant forms of TB, malaria, gonorrhoea and many other diseases are emerging. Their allies, the disease-carrying insects, once bombarded by pesticides, have also learned to evade the chemical assault, and will help to carry some of these microbes into new environments.

Air travel and world trade will greatly assist this process. Our relentless encroaching on new territory, our destruction and transformation of environments and our increasingly dense human settlements will rob microbes of old habitats and hosts; it will also force them to adapt

133

to new circumstances and new hosts, which will doubtless include not only us, but the crops and creatures we depend on for food. In this age-old battle, our ultimate victory is far from certain. (Garret 1995)

If the sudden and vicious onslaught of AIDS has cured our complacency about infectious disease it will have done us a great service. Ideas about closing down the world's epidemiological nerve centre, the US Centers for Disease Control in Atlanta, were abruptly dropped as epidemic diseases again became a reality. The need to refine counter-strategies has become urgent. (Gallo 1991:321–325)

Like the 1918 influenza epidemic which came, killed and disappeared in a few months, the next epidemic may not give us the luxury of a long lead-time. We had better learn the lessons well this time round. We may well have to face a barrage of new microbes in the coming years. If the AIDS pandemic has been a fire-drill, it has shown us to be remarkably unprepared to meet such onslaughts.

BIBLIOGRAPHY

BOOKS

Aggleton, P., Davies, P. and Hart, G. (eds) 1990 *AIDS: Individual, Cultural and Policy Dimensions*. London: Falmer Press.

Aggleton, P., Davies, P. and Hart, G. (eds) 1992. *AIDS: Rights, Risk and Reason*. London: Falmer Press.

AIDS in the World: A global report. 1992. The Global AIDS policy coalition, edited by Mann, J., Tarantola, D.J.M. and Netter, T.W. (eds) Cambridge, Mass: Harvard University Press.

Altman, Dennis. 1986. *AIDS in the Mind of America*. Garden City, New York: Doubleday/Anchor.

Altman, Dennis. 1988. *Legitimation through disaster:* AIDS and the gay movement, *in* Fee and Fox: 301–315.

Anderson, Roy M. and May, Robert M. 1992. 'Understanding the AIDS Pandemic'. *Scientific American* (May): 20–26.

Aral, S. O. and Holmes, K.K. 1991. 'Sexually transmitted Diseases in the AIDS era'. *Scientific American* 264 (No. 2, February): 18–25.

Bayer, R. and Healton, C. 1989. 'Controlling AIDS in Cuba: the Logic of Quarantine'. *New England Journal of Medicine* 320 (No.15, 13 April).

Bayer, Ronald. 1991. AIDS in the future of reproductive freedom, *in* Nelkin, Parris Willis, 191–215.

Berger, Peter L. 1986. Epilogue, *in* Hunter, J.D. and Ainlay, S.C. (eds), *Making Sense of Modern Times:* Peter L. Berger and the Vision of Interpretive Sociology. London: Routledge Kegan Paul, 221–235.

Bosk, Charles L. and Frader, Joel E. 1991. AIDS and its impact on Medical Work: The Culture and Politics of the Shop Floor, *in* Nelkin, Willis and Parris (eds), 150–171.

Brandt, Allan M. 1987. *No Magic Bullet: A social history of Venereal disease in the United States since 1880.* (Expanded edition with a new chapter on AIDS. Original edition 1985) New York: Oxford University Press.

135

Brogan, Patrick. 1992. *World Conflicts: Why and Where they are happening.* 2nd edition. London: Bloomsbury.
Broomberg, Jonathan. 1993. Current Research on the Economic Impact of HIV/AIDS: A Review of the International and South African Literature, *in* Cross and Whiteside, 34–57.
Bronski, Michael. 1989. *Death and the Erotic Imagination, in* Carter and Watney, 219–228.

Carter, Erica and Watney, Simon (eds). 1989. *Taking Liberties: AIDS and Cultural Politics.* London: Serpent's Tail Press.
Centre for Health Policy. 1991. *AIDS in South Africa: the demographic and economic implications.* Johannesburg: Department of Community Health, Medical School, University of the Witwatersrand, (Paper No. 23, September).
Chirimuuta, R.C. and R.J. 1987. *AIDS, Africa and Racism.* Derbyshire: R. Chirimuuta, Bretby House.
Crewe, Mary. 1992. *AIDS in South Africa: The myth and the reality.* London: Penguin.
Crewe, Mary. 1993. 'Learning AIDS'. *Work in Progress* (December): 25–28.
Crosby, Alfred W. 1989. *America's Forgotten Pandemic: The influenza of 1918.* Cambridge: Cambridge University Press.
Cross, Sholto and Whiteside, A. (eds) 1993. *Facing up to AIDS.* London: St Martin's Press.

Daniel, Herbert and Parker, Richard. 1993. *Sexuality, Politics and AIDS in Brazil: In another World?* London: Falmer Press.
Department of Health and Social Security. 1988. *Problems Associated with AIDS: Response by the Government to the Third Report from the Social Services Committee Session 1986–87 (January).* London: Her Majesty's Stationery Office.
Desclaux, Alice. 1994.'Silence as a form of public health policy? Breastfeeding and the transmission of HIV'. *Sociétés d'Afrique & SIDA.* (No. 6, October): 2–4.
Dols, Michael W. 1977. *The Black Death in the Middle East.* Princeton, New Jersey: Princeton University Press.

Bibliography

Everatt, David and Milner, Susan. 1994. Youth, AIDS and the Future, *in* Everatt, David (ed.). *Creating a Future: Youth Policy for South Africa.* Johannesburg: Ravan Press, 6–35.

Farmer, Paul. 1990. 'Sending Sickness: Sorcery, Politics and Changing Concepts of AIDS in Rural Haiti'. *Medical Anthropology Quarterly* 4 (No. 1, March): 6–27.

Fee, E. and Fox, D.M. (eds) 1988. *AIDS: The Burdens of History.* Berkeley: University of California Press.

Feldman, Douglas A. (ed.) 1994. *Global AIDS Policy.* Westport, Connecticut: Bergin and Garvey.

Filgueras, Ana. 1992/3 Needs of Rio Street Children, *in Planned Parenthood Challenges.* London: International Planned Parenthood Federation.

FitzSimons, D.W. 1993. The Global Pandemic of AIDS, *in* Cross, S. and Whiteside, A. (eds) 13–33.

Fleming, Alan. 1993. Lessons from tropical Africa for addressing the HIV / AIDS epidemic in South Africa, *in* Cross, S. and Whiteside, A. (eds) 295–317.

Foreman, M. and Taylor, J. with Claw, J. 1990. *The Third Epidemic: Repercussions of the Fear of AIDS.* London: Panos Institute.

Fox, Daniel M. 1988. The Politics of Physicians' Responsibility in Epidemics: A Note on History, *in* Fee and Fox, 86–96.

Fox, R.C., Aiken, L.H. and Messikomer, C.M. 1991. The Culture of Caring: AIDS and the nursing profession, *in* Nelkin, Willis and Parris, 119–149.

Freeman, R. 1992. The Politics of AIDS in Britain and Germany, *in* Aggleton, P. *et al* . (eds).

Gallo, Robert. 1991. *Virus Hunting: AIDS, Cancer and the human retrovirus – A story of scientific discovery.* New York: Basic Books.

Garrett, Laurie. 1995. *The Coming Plague.* New York: Farrar Strauss Giroux.

Gil, Vincent E. 1994. Behind the Wall of China: AIDS Profile, AIDS policy, *in* Feldman, Douglas A. (ed.), 7–27.

Goldstein, Richard, 1989. AIDS and the Social Contract, *in* Carter and Watney, 81–94.

Goldstein, R. 1991. The Implicated and the Immune: Responses to AIDS in the Arts and Popular Culture, *in* Nelkin, Willis, Parris, *A Disease of Society,* 17–42.

Gottfried, Robert. 1983. *The Black Death: National and Human Disaster in Medieval Europe.* New York: Free Press.

Green, Reginald H. 1991. 'Politics, Power and Poverty: Health for all in 2000 in the Third World?' *Social Science and Medicine* 32 (No. 7): 745–755.

Grover, Jan Zita. 1989. Constitutional Symptoms, *in* Carter and Watney, 147–159.

Hessling, Angelika and Heckmann, W. (eds). 1993. *Inventory of Psycho–social and Behavioural AIDS/drug research throughout Europe.* Berlin: AIDS Zentrum im Bundesgesundheitsamt.

Holland, J., Ramazanoglu, C., Scott, S., Sharpe, S. and Thomson, R. 1992. Pressure, resistance and empowerment: Young women and the negotiation of safer sex, *in* Aggleton, P. *et al.* (eds).

Holleran, Andrew. 1988. *Ground Zero.* New York: Plume Books (Div. of Penguin).

Juárez, A.L. 1992/3 Gente Joven: Meeting Needs, *in Planned Parenthood Challenges.* London: International Planned Parenthood Federation.

Ketting, Evert. 1992/3. A Global Picture, *in Planned Parenthood Challenges: Sexual and Reproductive Health.* London: International Planned Parenthood Federation.

Klouda, Anthony. 1992. 'Shifting patterns in International financing for AIDS Programs'. *AIDS in the World*: 787–801.

Kobasa, S.C.O. 1991. AIDS volunteering: Links to the past and future prospects, *in* Nelkin, Parris, Willis, 172–188.

Kramer, Larry. 1990. *Reports from the Holocaust: The making of an AIDS activist.* London: Penguin.

Larson, Ann. 1990. 'The social epidemiology of Africa's AIDS epidemic'. *African Affairs* 89 (No. 354, January): 5–26.

Mann, Jonathan, Tarantola, D.J.M., and Netter, T.W. (eds) with the Global

Bibliography

AIDS Policy Coalition. 1992. *AIDS in the World: A Global Report.* Cambridge, Mass: Harvard University Press.

Mariasy, Judith and Thomas, Laura with Radlett, M. 1990b *Triple Jeopardy: Women and AIDS.* London: Panos Institute.

Mayer, Philip and Iona. 1970. Socialization by Peers: The youth organisation of the Red Xhosa, *in* Mayer, P. (ed.). *Socialization: the approach from Social Anthropology.* (ASA Monograph 8.) London: Tavistock, 159–189.

McNeill, W.H. 1985. *Plagues and Peoples.* 1st edition 1976. Middlesex: Penguin.

Mhloyi, Marvellous M. 1991. 'AIDS Transition in Southern Africa: Lessons to be learned'. *Progress* (Spring/Summer): 44–49.

Miller, Norman and Rockwell, Richard C. (eds). 1988. *AIDS in Africa: The Social and Policy impact.* Lewiston, New York: The Edwin Mellen Press.

Musto, David F. 1988. Quarantine and the problem of AIDS, *in* Fee and Fox, 67–85.

NACOSA. 1994. *A National AIDS Plan for South Africa 1994–1995* (July) National AIDS Convention of South Africa: Sunnyside 0132.

Nelkin, Dorothy, Willis, D.P. and Parris, S.V. 1991. *A Disease of Society: Cultural and Institutional Responses to AIDS.* Cambridge: Cambridge University Press.

Nelkin, D., Willis, D.P. and Parris, S.V. 1991. Introduction: A Disease of Society – Cultural and institutional Responses to AIDS, *in* Nelkin Willis Parris (eds) 1–14.

Nohl, J. 1961. *The Black Death: A Chronicle of the Plague compiled from contemporary sources.* (1st edition 1926.) London: Unwin Books.

Obbo, Christine. 1993. 'The predicament of 'AIDS Orphans''. *Sociétés d'Afrique & SIDA* (No. 2, October): 8–9.

O'Connor, Anthony. 1991. *Poverty in Africa: a geographical approach.* London: Belhaven Press.

Osborn, June. 1988. 'AIDS: Politics and Science'. *The New England Journal of Medicine* (18 February): 445.

Overberg, Kenneth R. (ed.) 1994. *AIDS: Ethics and Religion.* New York: Orbis.

Packard, Randall M. 1989. *Epidemiologists, Social Scientists and the Structure of Medical Research on AIDS in Africa*. African Studies Centre Working paper No. 137). African Studies Centre, Boston.

Packard, Randall M. and Epstein, P. 1991. 'Epidemiologists, Social Scientists and the Structure of Medical Research on AIDS in Africa'. *Social Science and Medicine* 33 (No. 7): 771–794 (with comments and discussion).

Panos Dossier. 1988. *AIDS and the Third World*. London: Panos Institute.

Panos Dossier. 1990[a]. *The Third Epidemic – repercussions of the fear of AIDS*. London: Panos Institute.

Panos Dossier. 1990[b]. *Triple Jeopardy: Women and AIDS*. London: Panos Institute.

Panos Institute. 1992. *HIV and Development* (From Information to Education Series) (No.1, Spring). Washington: Panos Institute.

Patton, Cindy. 1989. *The AIDS industry:* Construction of 'victims', 'volunteers' and 'experts', *in* Carter, Erica and Watney, Simon (eds).

Patton, Cindy. 1990. *Inventing AIDS*. New York: Routledge.

Pickering, H., Todd, J., Dunn, D. *et al.* 1992. 'Prostitutes and their Clients: A Gambian Survey'. *Social Science and Medicine* 34: 75–88.

Porter, Dorothy and Roy. 1988. The Enforcement of health: the British Debate, *in* Fee and Fox, 97–120.

Ramphele, Mamphela. 1994. South African Youth: Millstone or opportunity? *in Leading Edge*, (Issue 2, December). Cape Town: Independent Development Trust, 39–40.

Risse, Guenter B. 1988. Epidemics and History: Ecological Perspectives and Social Responses, *in* Fee and Fox, 33–66.

Rosenberg, Charles E. 1988. *Disease and Social Order in America: Perceptions and Expectations, in* Fee and Fox, 12–32.

Sabatier, Renée. 1988. *Blaming others: Prejudice, Race and Worldwide AIDS*. Philadelphia: New Society Publishers.

Sabatier, Renée. 1989. *AIDS and the Third World*. London: Panos Institute.

Sanders, David with Carver, Richard. 1985. *The Struggle for Health: Medicine and the Politics of Underdevelopment*. London: Macmillan Education.

Bibliography

Schoepf, B.G. waNkera, R., Schoepf, C., Engundu, W. and Ntsomo, P. 1988. AIDS and society in central Africa: A view from Zaire, *in* Miller N. and Rockwell, R.C. (eds), 211–235.

Seftel, David. 1988. 'AIDS and Apartheid: Double Trouble'. *Africa Report* (Nov–Dec): 17–22.

Shilts, Randy. 1987. *And the Band Played On: Politics, People, and the AIDS Epidemic.* New York: St Martin's Press.

Singer, M., Flores, C., Davison, L., Burke, G., Castillo, Z., Scanlon K. and Rivera, M. 1990. 'SIDA: The Economic, Social and Cultural Context of AIDS among Latinos'. *Medical Anthropology Quarterly* 4 (No. 1, March): 72–114.

Sontag, Susan. 1989. *AIDS and its metaphors.* London: Allen Lane: The Penguin Press.

South African Institute of Race Relations. 1994. *'Fast Facts: A Picture of the Population'.* (No. 9, September).

South African Institute of Race Relations. (SAIRR) *Race Relations Survey 1991/92; 1992/93; 1993/94.*

Stoddard, Tom. 1989. *Paradox and Paralysis:* An overview of the American Response to AIDS, *in* Carter and Watney, 95–106.

Stoddard, Thomas B. and Rieman, Walter. 1991. AIDS and the rights of the individual: Toward a more sophisticated understanding of discrimination, *in* Nelkin, Willis, Parris, 241–271.

Stone, Alan B. and Hitchcock, P.J. 1994. 'Vaginal microbicides for preventing the sexual transmission of HIV'. *AIDS* 8 (Suppl.1): S285–S293.

Straker, Gill. 1992. *Faces in the Revolution: The Psychological Effects of Violence on Township Youth in South Africa.* Cape Town: David Philip.

Swenson, Robert M. 1989. 'Plagues, History and AIDS'. *Dialogue* (No. 83, 1:89): 16–22.

Taverne, Bernard. 1994. 'Ethics and Communication strategy: Female circumcision and AIDS in Burkina Faso'. *Sociétés d'Afrique & SIDA* (No. 6, October): 5–6.

Tolley, G.S. and Thomas, V. (eds) 1987. *The Economics of Urbanization and Urban Policies in Developing Countries.* Washington, D.C.: The International Bank for Reconstruction and Development – A World Bank Symposium.

Toms, Ivan. 1990. 'AIDS in South Africa: Potential Decimation on the Eve of Liberation'. *Progress* (Fall / Winter): 13–16.

Tuchman, Barbara, W. 1987. *A Distant Mirror: the Calamitous 14th Century.* (1st edition 1978.) Harmondsworth, UK: Penguin edition.

Turshen, Meredeth (ed.) 1991. *Women and Health in Africa.* New Jersey: Africa World Press.

UNICEF. 1993[a]. *AIDS: The Second Decade – a focus on youth and women.* New York: United Nations Children's Fund.

UNICEF – WHO Joint Committee on Health Policy. 1993[b]. *'Prevention and Control of AIDS in women and children'.* (JCHP 29/93.13, February). Geneva.

van der Vliet, Virginia. 1984. *Staying Single: A Strategy against Poverty?* Carnegie Conference Paper No. 116. South African Labour and Development Research Unit, University of Cape Town.

van der Vliet, Virginia. 1991. Traditional Husbands, Modern Wives?: Constructing Marriages in a South African Township, *in* Spiegel, A.D. and McAllister, P.A. (eds), *Tradition and Transition in Southern Africa (African Studies* 50th Anniversary Volume) Volume 50: Nos 1 and 2: 219–241

van der Vliet, Virginia. 1994. Apartheid and the politics of AIDS, *in* Feldman, Douglas A. (ed.), 107–128.

Whitehead, Tony. 1989. *The Voluntary Sector: Five Years On, in* Carter and Watney.

Whiteside, Alan. 1993. The impact of AIDS on industry in Zimbabwe, *in* Cross, S. and Whiteside, A. (eds), 217–240.

Whiteside, Alan and FitzSimons, David. 1992. *'The AIDS epidemic: Economic, Political and Security Implications'.* Conflict Studies 251. London: Research Institute for the study of conflict and terrorism.

World Health Organization/Global Programme on AIDS. 1993. *Effective Approaches to AIDS prevention: Report of a meeting.* (Geneva 26–29 May 1992) Geneva: WHO.

Yeager, Rodger. 1988. Historical and ecological ramifications for AIDS in Eastern and Central Africa, *in* Miller and Rockwell, 71–83.

Bibliography

PERIODICALS / NEWSPAPERS
The Argus. Cape Town.
Epidemiological Comments. Pretoria, South Africa.
The Guardian. London.
Independent on Sunday. London.
New African. London.
Newsweek. New York.
Sociétés d'Afrique & SIDA. Bordeaux, France.
Southern Africa Political and Economic Monthly. Harare, Zimbabwe.
Sunday Times. London.
Time. New York.
WorldAIDS. Panos Institute, London.

GLOSSARY

ACT-UP	AIDS Coalition to Unleash Power
ASO	AIDS service organizations
AZT	zidovudine (antiretroviral drug)
CDC	Centers for Disease Control (USA)
FDA	Food and Drug Administration
GMHC	Gay Men's Health Crisis
GPA	Global Programme on AIDS (WHO)
HIV	Human immunodeficiency virus
IUD	Intra-uterine device
MMWR	Morbidity and Mortality Weekly Review
N-9	Nonoxynol-9 (spermicide)
NGO	Non-governmental organizations
NIH	National Institutes of Health (USA)
ODA	Official development assistance
PWA	Person / people-with-AIDS
SAIRR	South African Institute of Race Relations
STDs	Sexually transmitted diseases
TB	tuberculosis
UN	United Nations
US	United States of America
WHO	World Health Organization

INDEX

ACT-UP, 70
Africa, 3, 14, 17ff, 23, 34, 36, 57,
    60, 61, 79, 81, 84ff
African AIDS organizations, 58ff
African epidemic, 57ff
Africans, 29, 53, 63, 64
AIDS: adolescents and HIV infec-
    tion, 106-7; African epidem-
    ic, 57ff; African origin
    hypothesis, 58ff; appearance
    of, 3, 27, 54, 55, 58; breast-
    feeding, 93; care, 103; and
    behavioural change, 121ff;
    and children, 97, 106; effect
    on psyche of communities,
    25; conspiracy spread theo-
    ries, 54; coping strategies, 8;
    debate in new areas, 8-9;
    disease cohorts, 21-3; cost of
    medical care, 21-3; coun-
    selling, 124; demographic
    change, 20, 108-110; ecolo-
    gy of disease, 78ff, 118; eco-
    nomic impact, 21; education,
    76, 89, 124; funding, 5, 33ff,
    69, 70, 72, 130; epidemiolo-
    gy, 18ff; habitat, 79; health
    care, primary, 126; HIV cau-
    sation disputed, 60, 131; and
    homosexuality, 62, 66, 67,
    75; infection rate, 19, 71-2,
    73; latency period, 20-1;
    lessons learned from, 117ff;
    medical fight against, 8-9;
    and medical profession,
    127ff; microbicides, vaginal,
    104-5; model of causation,
    6, 119; modus operandi, 20;
    mother-child link, 55, 92-3;
    and role of nurses, 131-2;
    orphans, 110; paediatrics,
    21; pandemic, 2ff; politi-
    cization of, 30ff; pro-
    grammes, 4, 18, 34, 35, 41,
    105; power/powerlessness,
    132; cost-effective projects,
    124; prognancy, 91-2; con-
    dom use in prostitution, 98ff;
    and clandestine protection
    methods for women, 103-5;
    and religion, 42ff; research,
    37ff, 127; risk, 56-7, 90;
    and schools, 106; seropreva-
    lence, 79, 92, 118, 119;
    social solutions, 120ff;
    socio-economic factors, 7,
    77ff; span, 8; spermicides,
    104; spread of, 81-2; state
    policy on, 28; sterilization of
    retarded women, 96; stigma-
    tization, 7-8, 27, 52ff; test-
    ing, 6; transmission of, 3,
    21, 27, 55, 71, 79, 86, 88ff,
    92-93, 122-3, 124; and
    urbanization, 79, 83ff; vac-
    cines for, 120, 127; and
    women, 89ff, 93ff, 101ff,
    virucides, 125-6; and youth
    106, 115 *see also* HIV
African green monkey, 63

Index

Le Pen, Jean Marie, 56
Leviticus, biblical, 52
Liberation movements, black and
     homosexual, 1
Liberia, 81
Los Angeles, 17, 63, 65

Malaria, 23, 60, 133
Malawi, 19, 57, 83, 88, 91
Malaysia, 56
Mandela, President Nelson, 51
Marcos regime, Philippines, 113
Maternity, status of, 95
Measles, 28, 59, 86, 120
Mediterranean, 79
Merson, Michael, 105, 125
MEXFAM, 44, 45
Mexican Family Planning
     Association, 44
Mexico, 11, 44, 74, 75
Microbes, drug resistant, 133, 134
Middle East, 10, 16, 53, 81
Migration, 80-81
Milan, Archbishop of, 14th century,
     15
Military personnel, role in prostitu-
     tion industry, 99
Mitchell, Dr Janet, 95
Monkeys, African, 63
Montagnier, Luc, 37, 38
Morocco, 43
Mozambique, 81, 82, 83
Mumps, 59
Muslim fundamentalists, 53, 56
Mutoko, Nathaniel, 102

Namibia, 58, 81
National AIDS programmes, 34, 35
National AIDS Trust, UK, 32
National Centre for HIV Social
     Research, Macquarie
     University Sydney, 71
National Institutes of Health, 30, 37,
     38
National Party, Australia, 56
Neil, Prof James, 61
New African, 61, 102
*New*sweek, 38, 39, 125
New York, 6, 17, 22ff, 30, 65, 67
New York Times, 25-6
NGOs, 6, 8, 48
Niebuhr, Barthold, 10, 24
Nigeria, 44, 59, 94, 98
Ninth International Conference on
     AIDS, Berlin, 1993, 105, 125
Njenga, Revd Stephen, 47
Non-governmental organizations,
     see NGOs
Nonoxynol-9, 104
North America, 36
Nurses, role in AIDS care, 131-2

Office of AIDS Research, NIH, 38
Orphans, AIDS, 110
Outreach projects for youth, 115

Paedophiles, 14
Pakistan, 74
Panos Institute, 23
Papua New Guinea, 44, 45, 99

105, 109, 119ff; as AIDS
risk factor, 39
Street children, 110ff
Street Kids International, 47, 112
Sudan, 81, 82, 91
Sunday Times, 60, 131
Switzerland, 73
Syphilis, 2, 59, 102

Tanzania 19, 23, 40, 57, 83, 94, 108
Thailand, 98, 113
Thalidomide crisis, 130-1
Thatcher, Margaret, 2, 65, 72
Third World, 19, 22, 35, 77, 81, 85, 88
Three Mile Island, 131
Time, 2
Tourism and HIV testing, 6
Townships AIDS programme, South Africa, 49
Tuberculosis, 18, 23, 60, 86, 87, 120, 133
Tunisia, 43
Typhoid, 28, 83
Typhus, 86

Uganda, 8, 17, 18, 54, 57, 81, 125
UK, 53
UNICEF: 106, 116; UN Children's Fund, 110
University of Zimbabwe, 94
US Committee for Refugees, 81
US gay subculture in 1970s, 78
US Supreme Court, 65
USSR, 54, 62

Vaccines, 120
Vatican, the, 44
Victimization, 52ff
Vietnam War, 1, 83
Virucide, woman controlled, 125-6

West Germany, 73-4
WHO: 19, 40, 57, 58, 93; Global Programme on AIDS, 4, 18, 105
Women: empowerment of, 103; with HIV, 89ff; hostility towards in heterosexual epidemics, 102; poor health care and education for, 106; potential to negotiate, 101-2; right to control own body, 96, 97; risk factors for, 90ff

Yellow fever outbreak, Philadelphia, 1793, 129
Yemen, 43, 44
Youth: empowerment, 115-16; perception of risk, 108; scepticism, 53-4; subcultures, 107; as victims, 106

Zaire, 23, 40, 83, 91, 102
Zambia, 22, 83, 91, 121
Zimbabwe, 22, 23, 41, 57, 91, 102

ALSO AVAILABLE IN THE BRIEFINGS SERIES

RETREAT FROM THE MODERN – Humanism, Postmodernism and the Flight from Modernist Culture by N.J. Rengger

A short but entertaining *tour d'horizon* of the factions and theories competing for high ground in the so-called culture wars. Dr Rengger takes us confidently through the conflicting (but also sometimes overlapping) positions which constitute the Modernist debate – from the Enlightenment through to postmodernism, via high humanism, pluralism, multiculturalism and anti-humanism.

In a wide-ranging discussion Dr Rengger deals with the work of all the foremost contributors to the debate, from Pico della Mirandola and the Baron Condorcet to Adorno, Steiner, Rorty, Habermas, Heidegger, Foucault, Derrida, Said, Bloom, Fish and others. Anyone who wants or needs to know more about the meaning of terms such as structuralism, postmodernism or deconstruction will find this book an invaluable guide.

N.J. Rengger is Lecturer in Politics at the University of Bristol and has been appointed Reader in Political Theory and International Relations at the University of St Andrews. He has published widely in contemporary political theory, intellectual history, cultural theory and international ethics. His most recent book is *Political Theory, Modernity and Postmodernity: Beyond Enlightenment and Critique* (B Blackwell, 1995). He is currently working on the interrelationship of culture and responsibility in international ethics.

UK: £9.99 USA: $14.95 Original Paperback ISBN: 0 906097 29 0